Poverty and Child Health

Second edition

Nick Spencer
Professor of Child Health
Department of Applied Social Studies
School of Postgraduate Medical Education
University of Warwick

Director
Centre for Community and Social Paediatric Research

Foreword by
Sir Donald Acheson
Chairman
International Centre for Health and Society
Former Chief Medical Officer

Radcliffe Medical Press

© 2000 Nick Spencer

Radcliffe Medical Press Ltd
18 Marcham Road, Abingdon, Oxon OX14 1AA

First edition 1996

British Library Cataloguing in Publication Data

A catalogue record for this book is available from the British Library.

ISBN 1 85775 477 8

Typeset by Advance Typesetting, Long Hanborough, Oxon
Printed and bound by TJ International Ltd, Padstow, Cornwall

Contents

Foreword

All of us who are worried about the many problems now faced by children throughout the world will be glad to see the second edition of Professor Nick Spencer's comprehensive and authoritative text. The new edition is timely because the period of complacency which has for some years marred the British approach to child health is now happily at an end. Thus recently the Prime Minister himself has made a pledge to eliminate child poverty and no less than 13 of the British government's self-imposed *Opportunity for All* targets are aimed at the health, education and material welfare of children and young people.

Consideration of the United Kingdom's place in comparison with other countries of the European Union shows how deep our concern should be. According to a recent analysis by UNICEF, although the UK's record on child well being is not entirely black 'the overall picture provides much cause for concern, with the UK emerging as a serious contender for the title of worst place in Europe to be a child'. Thus in 1995/6, the proportion of children in the UK in poverty (34%) was the highest in all the countries of the EU.

The recent *Independent Inquiry into Inequalities in Health* took the view that because childhood is a critical and vulnerable stage where poor socio-economic circumstances have lasting effects, priority should be given to policies directed at the health of parents and children. Thus, follow up of successive samples of births has pointed to the crucial influence of early life on subsequent mental and physical health and development. The fact that the adverse outcomes of early deprivation

– for example, mental illness, short stature, obesity, delinquency and unemployment – cover a wide range carries an important message. It suggests that policies which reduce such early adverse influences may result in multiple benefits not only throughout the life course of that child but to the next generation.

In his conclusions Professor Spencer is right to emphasise that future efforts to improve health must go far beyond purely medical interventions and embrace a wide range of social and economic policies which favour the less well off, whether in the UK or elsewhere. There is need for a plan of action right across government in partnership with the professions and the voluntary sector, together with a research programme which explores the fundamental mechanisms whereby psychosocial inequalities and poverty influence health.

Sir Donald Acheson
Chairman, International Centre for Health and Society
University College, London
July 2000

Acknowledgements

It is difficult to put in words the debt I owe to Professor John Emery; his inspiration and constant encouragement persuaded me to look beyond hospital paediatrics and to begin to address the social determinants of child health. Like many other of today's community and social paediatricians, it was John who put me on the 'road to community paediatrics'. Sadly, John died in a tragic accident whilst this second edition was in preparation. I would like to dedicate the book to his memory. I also owe much to Professor Sir David Hull who took over as my mentor when I moved to an unorthodox research post in Nottingham. With his help and encouragement, I have reached far beyond my early aspirations to an interest in academic child health. Since joining the European Society of Social Paediatrics (ESSOP), I have been privileged to work with, and count among my friends, many of the leading figures of European Social Paediatrics, including Lennart Kohler, Michel Manciaux and Bengt Lindstrom, whose wealth of experience and insight has proved invaluable in developing my own view of the social influences on child health. Nearer home but equally influential has been my friendship and academic cooperation with Stuart Logan; one of the unsung heroes of academic community child health, Stuart's depth of knowledge of social epidemiology has proved vital to the development of my understanding of the causal mechanisms in the determination of childhood ill health. Hilary Graham, Norma Baldwin and other staff members at the Department of Applied Social Studies in the University of Warwick not only accepted me as a full member of the

Department but have helped me to clarify and broaden my thinking in the area of social divisions and health. My thanks go to the University of Warwick for giving me study leave to work on this book and to my secretary, Carmel Parrott, and the other staff at the School of Postgraduate Medical Education who have provided invaluable support and shielded me from administrative duties to allow me precious writing time.

Introduction

The relationship between poverty and ill health has been the subject of debate and interest for over a century. Childhood is one of the most vulnerable periods in the human life-cycle and the health of children might be expected to suffer most as a consequence of poverty and its associated privations.

Given the extent of evidence relating material deprivation and adverse child health outcomes, the need for a book with this relationship as its primary focus could be questioned.

However, despite the apparent aetiological importance of poverty as a determinant of child health and the wide range of evidence available, there are few texts specifically aimed at bringing together evidence from different sources and considering the implications for social policy and healthcare systems.

The focus of the debate on the aetiology of adverse health outcomes in developed countries has shifted to health-related behaviours such as smoking and diet. This shift, combined with the political shift towards economic liberalism, particularly in the UK and USA in the 1980s, has fostered the view that individual health-related behaviours and not poverty are now the most important determinants of health in children as well as adults. In developing countries, cultural and behavioural factors such as resistance to family planning and unhygienic food handling practices have been advanced as alternative explanations for ill health amongst poor families.

This aetiological debate, itself not new, has far-reaching health and social policy implications. If poverty is no longer seen as a major health determinant and health inequalities are thought to arise as a consequence of unhealthy patterns of individual behaviour, then financially hard-pressed governments have a justified argument for the further reduction of social support and welfare programmes, and primary preventive strategies would be concerned more with changing individual behaviour than with social and environmental change.

In the UK, until the change of government in 1997, the Conservative government denied the links between poverty and health. They instituted social policies based on increasing income inequality whilst maintaining that the apparent association between poverty and ill health related solely to the health-related behaviour of lower income groups. The influence of this view was evident in the *Health of the Nation* document which, in addition to failing to consider children as a key group in the nation's future health, concentrated on behavioural solutions to current public health concerns and ignored the influence of social and material disadvantage on health.[1] The change of government has brought a change of attitude to poverty and health: the Labour government has recognised the association and, as well as revising the overall government plan for the public health to reflect this recognition,[2] has pledged to eradicate child poverty within 20 years and produced plans for multisectoral interventions aimed at reducing health inequalities.[3] Concerns persist, however, on two fronts: first, many of the proposed interventions continue to be based on changing health behaviour among individuals, and second, the pledges to reduce poverty are not accompanied by taxation policies aimed at reversing the gross inequalities in income distribution bequeathed by the previous administration.

The Acheson Report,[4] published 18 years after the Black Report,[5] reaches similar conclusions, linking material disadvantage directly to ill health. Recent work examining the links between early fetal and childhood experience and mortality in adult life, and longitudinal data tracing health experience throughout childhood amongst birth cohorts, has contributed to an understanding of the mechanisms by which material disadvantage may influence adverse health outcomes throughout the life course.[6–10] Based on this recent work, the Acheson Report[4] lays great emphasis on reducing material disadvantage among mothers and children stating:

> *We take the view that, while there are many poten-*
> *tially beneficial interventions to reduce inequalities*
> *in health in adults of working age and older people,*
> *many of those with the best chance of reducing future*
> *inequalities in mental and physical health, relate to*
> *parents, particularly present and future mothers and*
> *children.*

On the international arena, the debate has progressed beyond the level reached in the UK. The UN Convention on the Rights of the Child, eventually signed by the UK Government, and the WHO Health For All 2000 initiative formally recognise the rights of children to a standard of living adequate for their proper physical and mental development and specifically target the reduction of health inequalities. However, the targets are couched in general terms and do not address the social, political and medical problems of reducing health inequalities.

This book sets out to take a comprehensive view of poverty and child health, calling on evidence from a variety of sources, countries and historical periods. The second edition includes new material, bringing the book up to date, and new policy initiatives introduced by the UK Labour government to tackle health inequalities (in Part Four). Reviewers of the 1996 edition drew attention to some editing deficiencies; these have been rectified in this revised edition. In Part One, there are two chapters dealing with definition, measurement and extent of child poverty in the UK, Europe and the rest of the world. Also in this section is a chapter discussing the child health outcome measures against which the effects of poverty can be tested. Part Two deals with evidence from various sources linking poverty and child health; historical evidence particularly from the UK, evidence from less developed countries and evidence from developed countries. Part Three considers the causal debate and the mechanisms by which poverty and child health might be linked. Also included in this section is a chapter considering the relation between 'race', ethnicity, poverty and child health.

Part Four is concerned with future research studies, strategies for reducing health inequalities and the health and social policy implications of the conclusions from re-examination of the evidence.

The concluding chapter brings together the main points from each section focusing particularly on the continuity of evidence across countries and historical periods linking poverty and child health.

References

1   Department of Health (1992) *The Health of the Nation: A Strategy for Health in England*. HMSO, London.

2   Department of Health (1998) *Our Healthier Nation: A New Contract for Health*. The Stationery Office, London.

3   Department of Health (1999) *Reducing Health Inequalities: An Action Report*. Department of Health, London.

4   Department of Health (1998) *Independent Inquiry into Inequalities in Health (The Acheson Report)*. The Stationery Office, London.

5   Townsend P and Davidson N (1982) *Inequalities in Health: The Black Report*. Penguin, Harmondsworth.

6   Smith GD, Blane D and Bartley M (1994) Explanations of socio-economic differences in mortality: evidence from Britain and elsewhere. *Eur. J. Public Health*. 4:131–44.

7   Barker DJP (1992) *Fetal and Infant Origins of Adult Disease*. BMJ Publications Group, London.

8   Wadsworth MEJ (1991) *The Imprint of Time*. Clarendon Press, Oxford.

9   Power C, Manor O and Fox J (1991) *Health and Class: The Early Years*. Chapman & Hall, London.

10 Marmot M and Wilkinson RG (eds) (1999) *Social Determinants of Health*. Oxford University Press, Oxford.

To my grandfather, William Cloke, whose life taught me
the importance of the struggle for social justice
and education.

To my granddaughter, Charlotte Spencer-Jackson,
and my grandson, Luis Spencer-Parmakis, that they may,
in turn, learn from me.

To the memory of my friend and mentor,
Professor John Emery.

Part One

Definition and measurement

Defining and measuring poverty

This chapter is not intended as an exhaustive review of the long-running debate surrounding the definition and measurement of poverty. I have considered the essentials of the debate because of its importance in establishing the continued existence of poverty in developed countries and in giving a new impetus to the exploration of the effects of poverty on health. It also serves to warn the reader of some of the pitfalls inherent in defining and measuring poverty. In the brief review of approaches to measurement I have considered the profusion of measures of poverty, deprivation and socio-economic status used in government and international statistics and in health studies so as to inform subsequent chapters (Part Two) which consider the evidence linking poverty and child health and the causal debate (Part Three).

Defining poverty

'Absolute' and 'relative' poverty

There is broad acceptance that millions of people in less developed countries suffer levels of poverty which threaten their very existence. In the 19th century, Chadwick in Britain and Villerme in France documented similar desperate poverty in the burgeoning cities of the Industrial Revolution.[1,2] Such poverty can be characterised as 'absolute' in that those who suffer it have insufficient resources to sustain life and the health consequences are devastating (*see* Chapters 4 and 5).

The rise in living standards consequent upon dramatic economic expansion has all but eliminated absolute poverty in developed countries. However, substantial minorities in most developed countries have material resources insufficient to enable them to participate fully in the life of the societies to which they belong. Lack of resources imposes limits on housing, nutrition and leisure choices and they must forgo goods and services seen as 'necessities' by their fellow citizens.[3,4] Though not absolute in that their resources are adequate to sustain existence on a daily basis, their poverty can be described as 'relative'; relative, that is, to the living standards enjoyed by their fellow citizens.

Relative poverty is not a universally accepted concept. It has been challenged on the grounds that it merely identifies the less well-off and that, by using the definition in an extremely wealthy society, it would be possible to argue that inability to afford a new car every year would constitute poverty.[5]

In practice, as Alcock points out, any attempt to define a poverty line must include both relative and absolute elements.[6] It must change over time and be sensitive to 'necessities' of life in the specific society at the same time as establishing an absolute cut-off point below which poverty is said to exist. As early as the 1880s this was accepted by Booth, one of the early pioneers of poverty studies, who defined the very poor as those whose means were insufficient 'according to the normal standards of life in this country'.[7] Rowntree, in related studies of poverty in York (UK), though attempting to define an absolute subsistence level of poverty – including expenditure exclusively on minimum necessities to maintain merely physical efficiency – tacitly conceded that 'man (and more especially English man) cannot live by bread alone' when he included in his original measure expenditure on tea and modified his measure for the later studies to include expenditure on such items as a radio and books.[8,9]

Defining poverty lines

Most developed countries use an income 'cut-off' point as the poverty line. The European Union's (EU) poverty measure is below 50% of the national average income. The official poverty line in the USA uses income cut-offs which vary by family size.[10] As an alternative to income cut-off points, average expenditure devoted to necessities has been proposed as a means of determining the poverty level.[11]

In the UK, successive governments have resisted the pressure to define an official poverty line, reflecting in part a desire to minimise the extent of poverty in the UK and deflect criticism of social policy.[6] A vigorous debate has ensued which has included a reassessment of the effects of poverty on health and a renewed interest in health inequalities.[4,12]

Hidden poverty and 'double jeopardy'

The poverty definitions considered above, based on household incomes, do not account for uneven income distribution within a household leading to poverty which is 'invisible', nor do they account for the 'double jeopardy' experienced by ethnic minority groups in which poverty is created by, or exacerbated by, discrimination, overt or covert.

Women and children are the main victims of hidden poverty.[13] In households in which the family resources are earned and controlled by the man and women are given 'housekeeping' money, maldistribution has been shown to occur, leading to reduction in the food and fuel consumption of women and children within the family.[14] Women separated from their partners have reported that their financial situation improved after separation despite reliance on state benefits.[14]

The poverty experience of women and children has been further exacerbated by restrictions in public welfare services which have been a feature of government policy in the USA and most European countries in the last few decades. Women and children are the main beneficiaries of these services and they experience their loss more acutely. These restrictions impose a further burden on women, who undertake most caring roles within the family for children and other dependants.[15]

The relationship between race, ethnicity, poverty and child health is considered in detail in Chapter 7, and the specific effects of double jeopardy are explored. Suffice it to say here that the poverty experience of most ethnic minority groups is greater than that of the indigenous population as a result of discrimination and, for those in poverty, discrimination and racism ensure that their passage out is blocked.[10,16]

Hidden poverty and double jeopardy are not part of official definitions of poverty in developed countries. When considering the effects of poverty on child health both these factors need to be given special attention as children are likely to be disproportionately affected. In this book, wherever possible, I have drawn on evidence which addresses these important but poorly recognised aspects of the overall poverty experience of children.

The international dimensions of poverty

Though much of the evidence related to poverty and child health in this book is presented with reference to particular countries, it is important to recognise that poverty is an international phenomenon influenced by transnational as much as national economic and social policy and development.[4] Common elements can be identified despite the diversity of experience in different countries and the multiple influences of culture and tradition which mould poverty experience in individual countries.

These common elements include material disadvantage, powerlessness and exclusion from consumption either of the basic necessities of life or the goods and services which have become necessities within a particular society. Definition based on these common elements and enabling accurate comparison between countries is problematic.[4,6] However, for the purposes of this book, the common elements make it possible to use evidence of the effects of poverty on child health across many different cultures and countries to draw conclusions applicable to all children (*see* Part Four).

The international dimension of poverty goes beyond the problems and possibilities of definition. National economies are inextricably bound into an international economy and their place within this international economy has a significant influence on the extent of poverty within them as well as on the health and social policies they are able to pursue. It has been argued that the dramatic economic development of some countries, with the consequent disappearance of absolute poverty within their national boundaries, has taken place at the expense of other countries whose local economies have been destroyed, creating rather than alleviating poverty.[4,17] The debt crisis afflicting many less developed countries demonstrates the power of transnational economic interests to undermine the efforts of individual countries to alleviate poverty; it is the children already living in poverty in these countries who suffer most as a consequence (*see* Chapter 5).[18-20]

Low income, material disadvantage, deprivation and poverty

These terms are often used interchangeably. However, their meanings and the significance given to them require that some distinction is made. This will also help clarify the use made of the terms in this book.

- *Low income* describes those individuals, families or households whose regular income is low relative to others in the same country.

- *Material disadvantage* refers to those in a country whose material resources are limited to the extent that they are disadvantaged in their access to goods and services.

- *Deprivation* arises as a result of differential access to goods and services; deprivation is sometimes referred to as 'social', 'material' or 'multiple'.

- *Poverty* is an emotive term which is closely related to and encompasses all the preceding terms; poverty is never neutral and implies action to alleviate or eliminate it.[6]

In this book I have attempted to use these terms consistently and appropriately. The variety and range of sources used in the book have had an inevitable effect on my ability to stick to this good intention; however, I have adhered to it wherever possible. Poverty is chosen for the title consciously and deliberately, precisely because it goes beyond a neutral objective analysis and carries the implication of the need for action. In other words, this book not only describes the effects of poverty on child health but also considers and advocates approaches to the alleviation and reduction of these effects.

Measuring poverty

The problems of definition considered above are accompanied inevitably by problems of measurement. These are further compounded by the fact that some measures are applicable mainly to populations and others mainly to individuals within a population. In addition, measures may be specific to countries or groups of countries; for example, income proxies such as car ownership – which have been shown to be valuable measures in the UK – would be valueless in Bangladesh and, conversely, ownership of a small plot of land – a useful income proxy in Bangladesh – would have little or no relevance to the largely urbanised population of the UK.

It is clear that it is impossible to devise a single measure of poverty with international applicability. Here, I have reviewed available measures and commented on their usefulness and appropriate applications.

National and international 'poverty lines'

As discussed above, most countries have adopted an absolute poverty line based on income which, in practice, changes over time thus incorporating elements of the concept of relative poverty.

 In EU countries the measure is based on those households with incomes less than 50% of the average national income, though in some EU publications a measure based on 50% of average expenditure is used. Figures for Sweden quote a 'poverty line' of less than 58% of average equivalent disposable income.

Japan, Canada, Australia and the USA use a poverty measure which is kept constant over time in real terms; in other words, it does not vary with average income.[21] The US poverty lines are determined using a set of income cut-offs which vary by family size (in 2000, they ranged from $11 250 for two persons to $17 050 for a family of four to $28 650 for a family of eight (for each additional person add $2900)).[10] They have been used consistently for over 25 years and are adjusted annually to account for price increases. Adjustment for prices rather than incomes has led to a decline in the percentage of average income represented by the poverty lines; for example, the line for a family of four was about 43% of the median for all families in 1967, compared to 38% in 1988.[10]

The measures considered above are specific to countries and cannot be used for direct international comparison. However, their use is legitimate in comparing poverty trends over time between countries if the within-country measures remain constant (see Chapter 2). The problems of using cross-national poverty measures are illustrated in Figure 1.1, which shows the different distributions of poverty within EU countries when national and EU-wide poverty lines are used. This merely reflects the fact that incomes are unevenly distributed across the EU, with the result that the EU poverty line (50% of average EU income) in 1985 was two-thirds of the national average in a country such as Spain.[6]

In an attempt to develop comparable international income and poverty data, the government of Luxembourg has supported the development of an international database, known as the Luxembourg Income Study (LIS).[22] Data are collected on a recurrent basis from a number of advanced industrial countries and are adapted to give some measure of compatibility. Data from the LIS are considered further in Chapter 2.

National poverty lines are most often used to estimate the extent of, and trends in, poverty within countries. As such they are usually applied to populations and not individuals; however, they can be used in studies in which data are collected from individuals. The US poverty lines have been used extensively for this purpose.

a

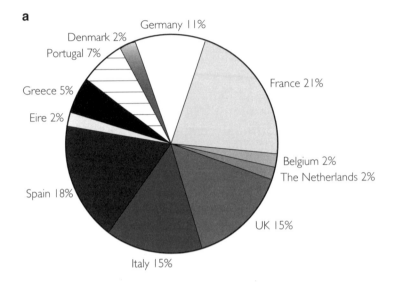

b

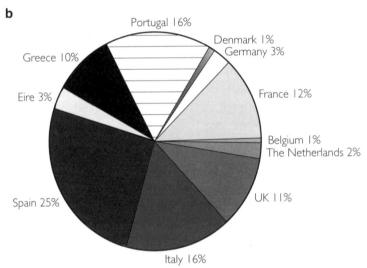

Figure 1.1   Distribution of poverty in Europe: (**a**) using national poverty lines; (**b**) using community-wide poverty lines. (Source [6] p. 43)

National and international measures of income inequality

Income inequalities occur in all countries and, as discussed above, this fact has been stressed in the argument against measures of relative poverty. Measures of the degree of income inequality within a country can be used to compare countries and characterise the gap between rich and poor within a country, providing a proxy measure of the extent of relative poverty.

A graphic example of the scale of income inequality is provided by Pen's 'Parade of Dwarfs'.[23] He represented individual share of overall income and resources by individual height, with average height equivalent to average income, and, in an imaginary hour-long parade of all British people, showed that it would be necessary to wait until 12 minutes before the end of the hour before persons of average height would pass by. In the last ten minutes of the hour giants would start to appear, with the tallest being over a mile high. Figure 1.2 shows the 'Parade' in diagrammatic form. A further striking example of the extent of inequality is the wealth of three Americans – Bill Gates, Warren Buffet and John Walton – whose combined

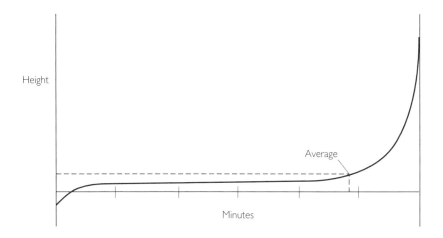

Figure 1.2   Pen's 'Parade of Dwarfs'. (Source [6] p. 110)

personal assets (US$94 billion) are greater than those of the
100 million poorest Americans.

Thus, the more unequal the income distribution within a
country, the more people there are living with incomes below
the average. A more scientific, if somewhat drier, representation
of income inequality is provided by Gini coefficients, which are
derived from Lorenz curves.[24] A Lorenz curve for a country
represents the actual income distribution against a hypothetical
distribution of completely identical incomes; in Figure 1.3, the
straight line is the hypothetical line of identical incomes and
the curved line is the line of actual incomes.

The Gini coefficient is derived by dividing the area between
the diagonal (line of identical incomes) and the curve (line of
actual incomes), the shaded area in Figure 1.3, by the total area
under the diagonal (line of identical incomes). Thus, the nearer
the Gini coefficient is to unity, the more unequal the income
distribution in the country.

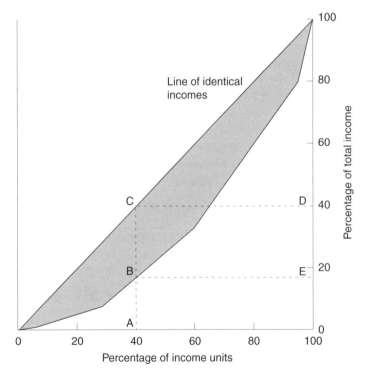

Figure 1.3   The Lorenz curve. (Source [6] p. 111)

Though useful for comparing income inequality between countries and trends in income distribution within countries over time, Gini coefficients are not widely estimated by governments themselves and are of no value in measuring the income levels of individual citizens or families.

Consensus or 'subjective' poverty measures

As discussed above, measures of relative poverty accurately reflecting the changing necessities of life within a particular society have proved difficult to devise. Most official and unofficial poverty lines constitute crude approximations of income levels, below which individuals and families are excluded from the necessities of life within a society. A novel and interesting approach to this problem has been the use of consensus or subjective measures based on the opinions of representative samples of the population.

Mack and Lansley, working with the commercial opinion polling company MORI and London Weekend Television, interviewed a representative UK sample of 1174 people.[3] Respondents were asked to list 'necessities of life' in contemporary Britain and to indicate whether they themselves had access to these necessities. An initial list of 26 items was identified which, in the opinion of more than 50% of respondents, constituted necessities. From this initial list, a composite list of 18 items of adult necessities and 18 items of child necessities was constructed, and an estimate made of those in the sample with no access to one or more of these items because of lack of resources rather than choice. From their data, the authors were able to estimate numbers of adults and children living in poverty and make an estimate of those living in extreme poverty, defined as those adults or children with no access to seven or more of the list of items because of lack of resources.

This approach has the advantage of easy repeatability in order to measure change in perception of necessity as well as change in the level of poverty as defined by this technique. London Weekend Television repeated the survey in the early 1990s; the results of both these surveys are considered further in Chapter 2.[25]

Townsend studied the opinions of a representative sample of 2700 adult Londoners between 1985 and 1986 on the levels of disposable income which they regarded as adequate for ordinary life and work.[4] In the opinion of the sample, the levels of adequate income by different family type were on average 60% higher than the means-tested state benefits for which such family types would be eligible. Using discriminant analysis of detailed income and deprivation data from the study, a threshold of necessary income to surmount poverty in different family types was calculated which, like the subjective data from the same study, suggested that state benefits were approximately 60% below the level of income required to surmount poverty.

A childhood poverty measure, the Children's Breadline Britain Index, based on asking parents which of a list of 32 items and activities they believed to be necessary for children in Britain to have in the early 1990s, has been developed.[26] Twenty-one of the items were seen as necessities by more than 50% of the parents of 1239 children included in the survey.

Consensus or subjective poverty measures can be used to measure levels of poverty as defined by the population, and as such are a closer approximation to relative poverty than the arbitrarily decided official poverty lines. As Townsend has demonstrated, they can be used to challenge official measures.[4] These measures are not developed or available in many countries so their use in international comparison is limited at present. Within countries they could be used in studies as measures of individual experience of deprivation.

Ecological measures of poverty and deprivation

Economic, health and education status measures of nation states, such as gross national product (GNP) and levels of female literacy, have been used as proxy measures for poverty and deprivation on an international level. These are a crude form of ecological measure in that they are applied to a population within a defined geographical area. Such measures can also be applied to regions of countries.

In this section we are more concerned with the development of within-country ecological measures of poverty and deprivation. In one of the earliest studies of the effects of poverty on health, Villerme classified areas of Paris according to rent rebate and demonstrated a clear gradient of mortality from the poorest to the most privileged.[2] In his study of poverty in the 1880s in London, Booth coloured streets on a map according to their level of poverty.[7] More sophisticated deprivation indices based on the socio-demographic characteristics of defined geographical areas have been devised in recent years and used in a number of countries.

A variety of socio-demographic indicators have been used to make up the deprivation indices and many are based on Census data. In the UK, where deprivation indices are widely used for health and local authority service planning and research, there has been an extensive discussion on the area indicators which most accurately reflect deprivation.[4,27] Deprivation indices developed by some government departments and by researchers interested in the influence of deprivation on primary healthcare have included indicators of demographic change as well as indicators reflecting material deprivation.[28]

The UK Department of the Environment produced the following list of eight indicators of urban deprivation:[29]

1   percentage of economically active persons who are unemployed

2   percentage of households defined as overcrowded

3   percentage of households with a single-parent family

4   percentage of pensioners living alone

5   percentage of households lacking exclusive use of two basic amenities

6   percentage of population change

7   standardised mortality rate

8   percentage of households in which the head was born in the New Commonwealth or Pakistan (a measure of recent immigration).

Jarman, using a more scientific method but incorporating a similar mixture of indicators, devised an eight-item weighted score which has been widely used in the allocation of resources to family health practitioners in the UK.[28] The weighting given to each item appears in brackets:

1   percentage of elderly living alone (6.62)

2   percentage of population aged under five (4.64)

3   percentage of lone-parent families (3.01)

4   percentage in social class V (3.74)

5   percentage unemployed (3.34)

6   percentage overcrowded (2.88)

7   percentage changing address within the past year (2.68)

8   percentage of ethnic minorities (2.50).

These indices have been criticised on the grounds that the combination of mainly demographic indicators, such as percentage of elderly and ethnic minorities, and indicators reflecting material deprivation, such as percentage of unemployed, represents a confusion over the nature of deprivation and a dilution of the influence of material deprivation.[4] Townsend points out that, as a consequence of this confusion, the indices fail to identify some of the most deprived areas of the UK.

An alternative approach has been to concentrate on those indicators which can be directly related to material deprivation.[30,31] The Townsend Deprivation Index defines material deprivation in terms of the following indicators, which are combined to give a score:[30]

1   percentage of those of economically active age who are unemployed

2   percentage of households which are overcrowded

3   percentage of households lacking a car

4   percentage of households not being buyers or owners.

A specific problem for all deprivation indices is the geographical unit to which the indicators apply. In the UK, Census data are built up from small enumeration districts (EDs) comprising approximately 100 households and aggregated into electoral ward data. Electoral ward data have been used in many studies of the effects of deprivation. However, electoral wards are often socially heterogeneous, with a mixture of deprived and non-deprived areas within them, thus diluting and distorting the extent of deprivation. To surmount this problem, aggregated ED data ranked according to deprivation scores have been used.[32] Using this approach, it is possible to compare the most deprived aggregated decile of EDs with the least deprived decile (*see* Chapter 6). An alternative use of EDs is to aggregate adjacent EDs with similar deprivation and age-group characteristics into homogeneous social areas. This method has been used to study the social patterning of accident rates in preschool children.[33]

A further criticism of ecological measures, especially when applied in the UK context, is that they fail to adequately reflect rural poverty. Gordon[34] derived a measure of child poverty in a rural area of the UK (Somerset) based on census variables which had also been shown to be strongly related to child poverty in deprivation surveys.[3,25] Six variables, all related to households with dependent children, were included in the measure. The weighting given to each item appears in brackets:

1   no earners – no adult in employment (39.5%)

2   renters – rented accommodation (21.4%)

3   overcrowding – more than one person per room (18.1%)

4   lone parent – dependent children and only one adult (6.9%)

5   no car – no access to car (6.7%)

6   no heat – no central heating (6.4%).

Applying this measure in the rural county of Somerset, Gordon reports less of an urban bias than other measures of child poverty and other generic deprivation indices.[34]

Similar indices of deprivation have been used in other countries such as Spain and the USA.[35,36]

Ecologically-based deprivation indices have distinct advantages:

- census data are widely available, at least in most developed countries

- data on income and other indicators of deprivation do not have to be collected again from individual households for each study

- they enable planning and targeting of resources and provide a measure of social need

- the address of an individual can be used as a proxy for material deprivation

- they provide a ready means of comparing areas and regions in relation to deprivation experience.

Indices have not been standardised across national borders and are specific to the society in which they are developed. As indicated above, caution must be employed in their use and interpretation, especially when they are applied to heterogeneous areas. The choice of indicators used needs to be closely related to the purpose of study being undertaken and it would seem advisable to avoid indices based on a mixture of indicators related to different aspects of deprivation.

Measures of income, income proxies and socio-economic status (SES)

Though not strictly measures of poverty, it is on these measures that much of the evidence for health inequalities is based as they have been extensively employed in socio-medical research in many different countries (*see* Chapters 5 and 6). Whilst not measuring all the dimensions of poverty, their use is legitimate in the study of the effects of poverty on health as most of them reflect income levels and official poverty measures are based on income (*see* above).

In many studies, particularly in the USA, income is used as the main measure of SES. In the USA this can be directly related to an income cut-off for family type and classified according to the official poverty lines. In the UK, there is little tradition of using income in socio-medical research and the absence of official poverty lines makes it difficult to classify income in terms of poverty. Research subjects have been classified as 'low income' or state benefit levels have been used to determine incomes below which individuals or households can be said to be living in poverty. Despite the reluctance to use direct income measures in socio-medical research, Townsend has demonstrated the possibility of obtaining detailed and extensive data related to income and financial resources in a representative sample of the UK population.[37]

A range of income proxy measures have been used either because data are readily available from other sources such as the Census or, as in the UK, to avoid direct income measures. Two such measures which have been increasingly used in the UK are car ownership and housing tenure (owner occupier or tenant). These have been shown to be closely related to disposable income and to discriminate better than social class for health outcomes.[38] Car ownership and housing tenure, though useful income proxies in the UK, do not necessarily have the same applicability to other developed countries; in France, for example, the majority of the population live in rented accommodation and housing tenure would not be a good discriminant. In many developed countries, level of parental education serves as a useful income proxy. In the USA, 'race' seems to be used in many studies as an income proxy – the significance of 'race' and poverty is discussed in Chapter 7.

Land ownership has been used as an income proxy in studies in rural areas of less developed countries such as Bangladesh. Maternal education and literacy levels have also been used, although they are less closely related to income.

Classifications of occupation have been extensively used as measures of SES. Perhaps the best known of these and the most influential in the debate on the health effects of poverty is the

Registrar General's Social Class (RGSC) used in official UK statistics and in many socio-medical studies. The RGSC, by which the occupation of the head of the household (usually taken to mean the husband) is classified into one of six groups (I, II, III non-manual, III manual, IV and V), was first introduced in the 1911 Census. Subsequently, the classification has been modified on a number of occasions.

The RGSC has been a powerful tool in identifying differences in health, education and many other aspects of life by SES and tracing those differences over time (*see* Chapter 6). Much of the impetus for the renewed debate on the effects of poverty on health, at least in the UK, arises from the Black Report on health inequalities, the data for which were derived mainly from official publications using the RGSC as the main SES measure.[39]

However, the RGSC, along with other classifications based on the occupation of the head of the household, has serious limitations which have been increasingly recognised in recent years. Social and demographic changes in most developed countries have ensured that many households have no male head; in the UK as many as 25% of babies are now born outside conventional marriages. Along with the steep rise in unemployment in many developed countries, these changes mean that an increasing minority of the population is 'unclassifiable' by the RGSC. Of particular importance in the study of the health effects of poverty is that these groups tend to be the most deprived, with the consequence that misleading conclusions can be drawn from statistics in which they are omitted or inadequately classified (*see* also Part Three).[40,41] For example, in studying the impact of social inequalities on birthweight, the RGSC has been shown to underestimate the impact when compared with an ecological measure which incorporates all births, including those to lone mothers.[42]

The focus of the RGSC on the male head of household has been criticised from a feminist perspective, particularly when it is being used to study SES differences that relate specifically to women and children.[43] Jones and Cameron have pointed out that the RGSC conceals many major intra-class variations in health outcomes.[44]

As a result of the shortcomings of the RGSC, many researchers have turned to income proxies (*see* above) such as car ownership and housing tenure.[38] Others have developed SES measures incorporating a number of socially related factors.[45,46] Canadian researchers have developed a more comprehensive measure of economic and social well-being, the Personal Security Index, which includes measures of perceived economic and physical security.[47]

A further dimension of poverty, directly related to measures of individual socio-economic status, is length of time in poverty. Studies based in the USA[48] and the UK[49] have included length of time in poverty as a variable, demonstrating that it is a more powerful predictor of adverse outcomes and adverse health behaviours (such as smoking) than simple measures of income or receipt of state benefits (*see* also Part Two).

This group of measures, because of their extensive use in socio-medical research, forms the basis of much of the evidence discussed in later chapters of this book. Results based upon them should be interpreted carefully, especially when considering the health effects of poverty rather than specifically low SES; however, treated with appropriate caution and considered alongside evidence derived using different measures, this vast body of evidence can throw light on the effects of poverty on child health. Their principal use is as measures of the SES of individuals or households. Their use in international comparisons is limited; income and occupational trends over time can be compared, as can national and regional maternal education and literacy levels.[50]

Qualitative measures

Poverty affects families and children rather than statistics! In the discussion of definitions and scientifically verifiable quantitative measures, this truism is frequently forgotten. Qualitative data, which give voice to those experiencing poverty, provide a dimension for understanding and exploring poverty and its consequences not available in purely quantitative research. The major UK poverty studies, from Booth and Rowntree through to Townsend, have included important qualitative data describing the reality of life in poverty.[7,9,37] Over time these provide interesting and important comparisons of changing patterns of poverty experience as well as bringing to life the otherwise rather dry statistics.

Qualitative research has succeeded in identifying previously hidden aspects of poverty, such as that discussed above associated with the maldistribution of income within families (p. 5). In the absence of good quantitative measures of hidden poverty and the double jeopardy of ethnic minorities, qualitative approaches remain the mainstay of measurement of these aspects of poverty.

Qualitative research has deepened our knowledge of ill-understood aspects of the poverty experience; for example, accounts of the nutritional privations associated with poverty collected in a series of mainly qualitative studies in the UK, and qualitative data on the reasons for the social gradient in women's smoking, have influenced the causal debate on the health effects of poverty (*see* Part Three), as well as carrying important implications for health promotion (*see* Part Four).[14,51,52]

Qualitative research is more difficult to standardise and the methodology of qualitative studies tends to be variable and disputed. Although validated methods exist and methodological rigour is as important as for quantitative research,[53] it lacks the precision and reproducibility required for national and international comparison. Its strength lies in substantiating quantitative data and in generating hypotheses and revealing previously unidentified aspects of the poverty experience.

Summary

1   Definitions of poverty are problematical though the research consensus favours a relative concept in developed countries.

2   Official poverty measures (poverty lines) are generally based on income and incorporate elements of both the relative and absolute concepts of poverty.

3   Gini coefficients, derived from Lorenz curves, provide a measure of income inequality within a country and a means of comparing countries based on income distribution.

4   Consensus or subjective poverty measures are a potential and, as yet, unproven solution to the problem of defining poverty lines which are truly relative and providing an alternative to the somewhat arbitrary official poverty lines.

5   Ecological measures of deprivation derived from Census data are increasingly used in service planning and in research, where they offer a readily available alternative to the collection of SES data from individuals or households.

6   Income, income proxies and SES measures are widely used in socio-medical research and, when used and interpreted with caution, provide a wealth of evidence of the health effects of poverty.

7   Qualitative measures are unstandardised but are the only measures available of certain types of poverty, such as hidden poverty, and have an important role in the identification and elucidation of ill-understood aspects of the experience of living in poverty.

References

1   Flinn MW (ed.) (1965) *Report on the Sanitary Conditions of the Labouring Population of Great Britain, by Edwin Chadwick, 1842*. Edinburgh University Press, Edinburgh.

2   Villerme LR (1826) Rapport fait par M. Villerme, et lu a l'Académie de Médicine, au nom de la Commission de Statistique, sur une série de tableaux rélatifs au mouvement de la population dans les douze arrondissements municipaux de la ville de Paris pendant les cinq années 1817–21. *Archives Générales de Médicine*. **10**:216–45.

3   Mack J and Lansley S (1984) *Poor Britain*. George Allen and Unwin, London.

4 Townsend P (1993) *The International Analysis of Poverty.* Harvester Wheatsheaf, Hemel Hempstead.

5 Sen AK (1983) Poor relatively speaking. *Oxford Economic Papers.* **35**:153–69.

6 Alcock P (1993) *Understanding Poverty.* Macmillan, London.

7 Booth C (1889) *Labour and Life of the People: Vol. 1, East London.* Williams and Norgate, London.

8 Rowntree BS (1901) *Poverty: A Study of Town Life.* Macmillan, London.

9 Rowntree BS (1941) *Poverty and Progress: A Second Social Survey of York.* Longman, London.

10 Danziger S and Stern J (1990) *The causes and consequences of child poverty in the United States.* Innocenti Occasional Papers, No. 10, Unicef International Child Development Centre, Florence, Italy.

11 Orshansky M (1969) How poverty is measured. *Monthly Labor Rev.* **92**:37–41.

12 Townsend P, Davidson N and Whitehead M (1992) *Inequalities in Health: The Black Report and The Health Divide.* Penguin, Harmondsworth.

13 Glendinning C and Millar J (1987) *Women and Poverty in Britain.* Harvester Wheatsheaf, Hemel Hempstead.

14 Graham H (1987) Women's smoking and family health. *Soc. Sci. Med.* **25**:47–56.

15 Graham H (1993) *Hardship and Health in Women's Lives.* Harvester Wheatsheaf, Hemel Hempstead.

16 Green P (1981) *The Pursuit of Inequality.* Pantheon Books, New York.

17 Navarro V (ed.) (1982) *Imperialism, Health and Medicine.* Pluto Press, London.

18 Godlee F (1993) Third world debt. *BMJ*. 307:1369–70.

19 Costello A, Watson F and Woodward D (1994) *Human Faces or Human Facade? Adjustment and the Health of Mothers and Children*. Centre for International Child Health, Institute of Child Health, London.

20 Sanders D (1985) *The Struggle for Health*. Macmillan Education, London.

21 Cornia GA (1990) *Child poverty and deprivation in industrialised countries: recent trends and policy options*. Innocenti Occasional Papers, No. 2, Unicef International Child Development Centre, Florence, Italy.

22 Smeeding TS, O'Higgins M, Rainwater L *et al.* (1990) *Poverty, Inequality and Income Distribution in Comparative Perspective*. Simon and Schuster, London.

23 Pen J (1971) A parade of dwarfs (and a few giants). In *Income Distribution* (ed. TS Preston). Penguin, Harmondsworth.

24 Atkinson AB (1983) *The Economics of Inequality* (2e) Oxford University Press, Oxford.

25 Mack J and Lansley S (1992) *Breadline Britain in the 1990s*. HarperCollins, London.

26 Middleton S, Ashworth K and Braithewaite I (1997) *Small Fortunes: Spending on Children, Childhood Poverty and Parental Sacrifice*. Joseph Rowntree Foundation, York.

27 Spencer NJ and Janes H (eds) (1992) *Uses and Abuses of Deprivation Indices: Report of a Conference at the University of Warwick*. School of Postgraduate Medical Education, University of Warwick, Coventry.

28 Jarman B (1983) Identification of underprivileged areas. *BMJ*. 289:1587–92.

29 Department of the Environment (1983) *Urban Deprivation*. Information Note Number 2, Inner Cities Directorate, Department of the Environment, London.

30 Townsend P, Phillimore P and Beattie A (1988) *Health and Deprivation*. Croom Helm, Beckenham.

31 Carstairs V (1981) Multiple deprivation and health state. *Community Med.* 3:4–13.

32 Reading R, Openshaw S and Jarvis SN (1990) Measuring child health inequalities using aggregations of enumeration districts. *J. Public Health Med.* 12:160–7.

33 Haynes R, Lovett A, Reading R *et al.* (1999) Use of homogeneous social areas for ecological analysis: a study of accident rates in preschool children. *Eur. J. Public Health.* 9:218–22.

34 Gordon D (1996) *Draft Report on Budget Allocation and Child Poverty in Somerset*. Statistical Monitoring Unit, School for Policy Studies, University of Bristol, Bristol.

35 Armero MJ, Frau MJ and Colomer C (1991) Health indicators for urban areas: geographic variation according to social coherence. *Gaceta Sanitaria* (Spanish). 22:17–20.

36 Valdes-Dapena M, Birle LJ, McGovern JA *et al.* (1968) Sudden unexpected death in infancy: a statistical analysis of certain socioeconomic factors. *J. Pediatr.* 73:387–94.

37 Townsend P (1979) *Poverty in the United Kingdom*. Penguin, Harmondsworth.

38 Smith GD, Blane D and Bartley M (1994) Explanations of socio-economic differences in mortality: evidence from Britain and elsewhere. *Eur. J. Public Health.* 4:131–44.

39 Townsend P and Davidson N (1982) *Inequalities in Health: The Black Report*. Penguin, Harmondsworth.

40 Pamuk ER (1988) Social class inequality in infant mortality in England and Wales from 1921 to 1980. *Eur. J. Popul.* 4:1–21.

41 Judge K and Benzeval M (1993) Health inequalities: new concerns about the children of single mothers. *BMJ.* 306: 677–80.

42 Spencer NJ, Bambang S, Logan S *et al.* (1999) Socio-economic status and birthweight: comparison of an area-based measure with the Registrar General's social class. *J. Epidemiol. Community Health.* 53:495–8.

43 Oakley A, Rigby AS and Hickey D (1993) Women and children last? Class, health and the role of maternal and child health services. *Eur. J. Public Health.* 3:220–6.

44 Jones IG and Cameron D (1984) Social class – an embarrassment to epidemiology. *Community Med.* 6:37–46.

45 Hollingshead AB and Redlich FC (1958) *Social Class and Mental Illness: A Community Study.* Wiley, New York.

46 Osborne AF (1987) Assessing the socioeconomic status of families. *Sociology.* 21:429–48.

47 Canadian Council on Social Development (1999) *Personal Security Index 1999.* Canadian Council on Social Development, Ottawa.

48 Duncan GJ, Brookes-Gunn J and Klebanov PK (1994) Economic deprivation and early childhood development. *Child Develop.* 65:296–318.

49 Graham H and Blackburn C (1998) The socio-economic patterning of health and smoking behaviour among mothers with young children on income support. *Sociol. Health and Illness.* 20:215–40.

50 Grant J (1994) *The State of the World's Children.* Oxford University Press, New York.

51 Lang T (1984) *Jam Tomorrow?* Food Policy Unit, Manchester Polytechnic, Manchester.

52 National Children's Home (1992) *Deep in Debt: A Survey of Problems Faced by Low Income Families.* NCH, London.

53 Mays N and Pope C (2000) Assessing quality in qualitative research. *BMJ.* 320:50–2.

2

The extent of child poverty

Introduction

Given the difficulties of definition and measurement outlined in Chapter 1, there are inevitable problems in the estimation of the extent of poverty. However, data are available from various sources which permit a reasonable estimate of the numbers of children living in poverty in various parts of the world. For the USA, the UK and some other European countries data on recent trends in childhood poverty are available; reliable data related to trends in less developed countries are not available but some estimate of poverty trends is possible.

In this chapter, I consider the global experience of child poverty and the striking differences in poverty experience of children in different parts of the world. Child poverty in the less developed world is then considered, followed by data from the USA and Europe, with a particular focus on the UK. The role of the debt crisis in increasing child poverty and exacerbating existing poverty in many less developed countries is considered, as are some of the reasons for increases in child poverty in some developed countries. The trend across all developed countries for children to replace the elderly as the most numerous age group in poverty is discussed.

The global experience of child poverty

Despite the doubling of the overall growth of the world economy in the 25 years up to 1998, an estimated 1.3 billion of the world's people lived in absolute poverty on less than US$1 per day in 1998.[1] The vast majority of those in absolute poverty live in low-income countries[2] and children make up the largest single group of those in poverty.

Women and children are most vulnerable to poverty, the most visible effect of which, in many countries, is malnutrition (*see* Chapter 5).[2] Based on 1975 data, Table 2.1 shows estimates of children affected by malnutrition in different continents.

The international maldistribution of poverty is not merely coincidental: the wealth of the rich countries depends in part on the continuing poverty of poor countries and helps to maintain low educational and income levels which benefit rich economies.[3,4] One way of representing this difference is to look at differential consumption levels between the developed and less developed worlds. The impact of the average citizen in the USA on the global environment in terms of consumption has been estimated at three times that of the average Italian, 13 times that of the average Brazilian, 35 times that of the average Indian, 140 times that of the average Bangladeshi and more than 250 times that of a citizen of one of the least developed nations of sub-Saharan Africa.[5] Also bear in mind that these are averages: in each country there are huge differences in access to consumption, with the inevitable consequence that the difference between the biggest consumers in the USA and the smallest consumers in sub-Saharan Africa will be even greater. In global terms, the rich nations are consuming four-fifths of the world's resources and the income disparity between the

Table 2.1   Total number of children affected by malnutrition by continent. (Source [2] p. 4)

Area	Population (millions) age 0–5 years	No. with malnutrition (millions)		
		Severe	*Moderate*	*Total*
Latin America	46	0.7	8.8	9.5
Africa	61	2.7	16.3	19.0
Asia	206	6.6	64.4	71.0
Grand total	314	10.0	89.5	99.5

richest and the poorest 20% of the world's population has doubled over the last 30 years.[6] The extent of the income disparity at a personal level is illustrated by the combined wealth of the world's richest 225 people, which is equivalent to the annual income of the poorest 2.5 billion (nearly half the world's population).[1]

The relation between rich industrial and less developed countries was unequal during the period of colonial rule when resources were drained from colonised areas into the colonising country. Since the end of colonial rule in most parts of the world, the unequal relationship has continued. Sanders highlights the role of multinational companies, which have incomes greater than the GNP of many countries.[7] Figure 2.1 illustrates this process by which resources continued to be drained from Latin America between 1960 and 1967. In 1992, partly as a result of the debt crisis (*see* Chapter 10, p. 285), there was a net flow of US$19 billion from the 40 poorest countries in the world to the richest.[8]

Child poverty in less developed countries

As indicated above, the bulk of the world's poor live in less developed countries. The demography of these countries ensures that the majority of their populations are young.[2,7] In the 1970s, there were estimated to be 500 million children under five years of age and 400 million of these lived in less developed countries.[7] Half of these 400 million under-fives live in absolute poverty and children in less developed countries are almost twice as likely to be poor as the population as a whole.[9] Children account for 43% of the Latin American and Caribbean populations living in poverty and, as Unicef states: 'most of the regions' children are poor and most of the poor are children'.[10]

In less developed countries poverty dominates in rural areas, though rapid urbanisation is creating new problems in terms of overcrowding and lack of environmental resources to sustain huge influxes of population. Seventy-seven per cent of those in absolute poverty in less developed countries live in rural areas.[9] Most are either small farmers or lease land or are landless

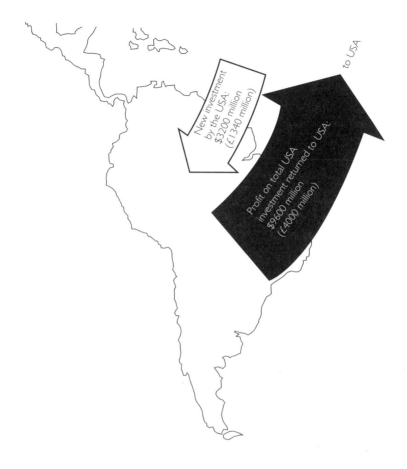

Figure 2.1   Inflow and outflow of capital from Latin American countries, 1960–67. (Source [7])

labourers who are found particularly in the high-population-density countries of the Indian subcontinent.[2] Many of the rural poor in these countries are caught in what has been described as the PPE (Poverty, Population, Environment) spiral.[5] The spiral is illustrated in Figure 2.2.

The spiral suggests that reduced educational, healthcare and sanitation opportunities as well as increased unemployment would tend towards acceleration of the spiral. The structural adjustment programmes (SAPs) introduced by the World Bank and the International Monetary Fund (IMF) have targeted

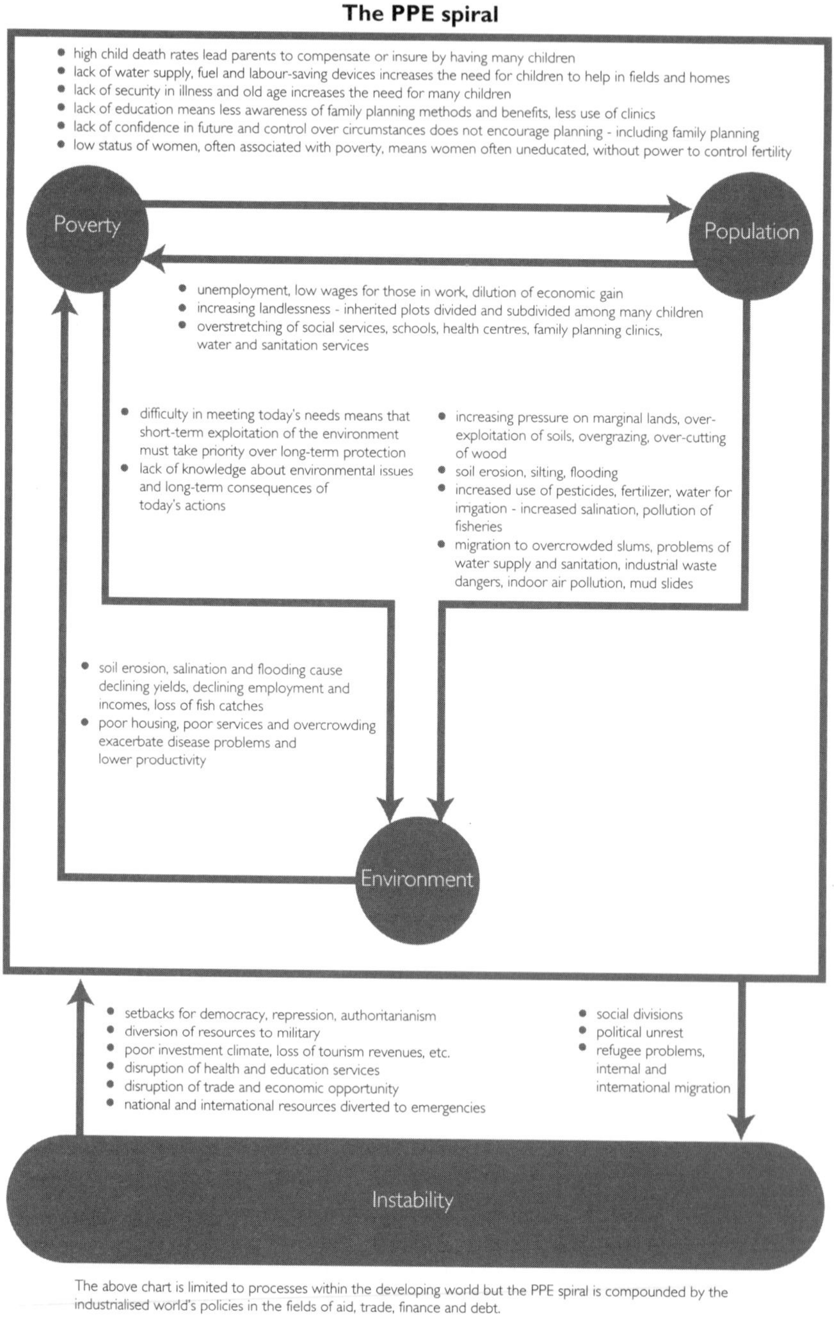

The PPE spiral

- high child death rates lead parents to compensate or insure by having many children
- lack of water supply, fuel and labour-saving devices increases the need for children to help in fields and homes
- lack of security in illness and old age increases the need for many children
- lack of education means less awareness of family planning methods and benefits, less use of clinics
- lack of confidence in future and control over circumstances does not encourage planning - including family planning
- low status of women, often associated with poverty, means women often uneducated, without power to control fertility

Poverty

Population

- unemployment, low wages for those in work, dilution of economic gain
- increasing landlessness - inherited plots divided and subdivided among many children
- overstretching of social services, schools, health centres, family planning clinics, water and sanitation services

- difficulty in meeting today's needs means that short-term exploitation of the environment must take priority over long-term protection
- lack of knowledge about environmental issues and long-term consequences of today's actions

- increasing pressure on marginal lands, over-exploitation of soils, overgrazing, over-cutting of wood
- soil erosion, silting, flooding
- increased use of pesticides, fertilizer, water for irrigation - increased salination, pollution of fisheries
- migration to overcrowded slums, problems of water supply and sanitation, industrial waste dangers, indoor air pollution, mud slides

- soil erosion, salination and flooding cause declining yields, declining employment and incomes, loss of fish catches
- poor housing, poor services and overcrowding exacerbate disease problems and lower productivity

Environment

- setbacks for democracy, repression, authoritarianism
- diversion of resources to military
- poor investment climate, loss of tourism revenues, etc.
- disruption of health and education services
- disruption of trade and economic opportunity
- national and international resources diverted to emergencies

- social divisions
- political unrest
- refugee problems, internal and international migration

Instability

The above chart is limited to processes within the developing world but the PPE spiral is compounded by the industrialised world's policies in the fields of aid, trade, finance and debt.

Figure 2.2 The poverty, population and environment (PPE) spiral. (Source [5])

expenditure by debtor governments on employment, wages, health services, education and welfare, but military expenditure seems to have been exempt.[8] As a result, for example, in Africa primary school enrolment of boys and girls fell between 1980 and 1990 by 7%.

However, poverty trends in less developed countries are disputed. The World Bank maintains that poverty has changed little in the late 1980s. Although the percentage of people in less developed countries living below the poverty line fell from 30.5% in 1985 to 29.7% in 1992, the actual number rose from 1.05 billion to 1.13 billion.[9,11] However, in some regions of the world much more marked increases were noted, in both absolute numbers and percentages: in sub-Saharan Africa from 184 (47.6%) to 216 million (47.8%); Middle East and North Africa from 60 (30.6%) to 73 million (33.1%); Latin America and the Caribbean from 87 (22.4%) to 108 million (25.5%). In South Asia, the percentage decreased from 51.8% to 49% but the numbers increased from 532 to 562 million.

Overall, it seems that poverty is increasing in many areas of the less developed world and children are its main victims. As suggested by Logie and Woodroffe, and Godlee, the SAPs enforced on many poor countries are likely to exacerbate and increase this trend and the programmes are wrongly targeted as they put in jeopardy the already precarious situation of many of the world's poor.[8,12]

Child poverty in developed countries

Given the magnitude and intensity of child poverty in less developed countries, it could be suggested that the relative poverty of 200 million people, including many children, in developed countries represents an insignificant part of the global burden of poverty. There is a direct and organic connection between poverty in less developed and developed countries which arises from the international nature of the world economy and its influence across national boundaries. Structural factors perpetuating and exacerbating poverty in Bangladesh can be seen to have an influence on poverty in the inner-city areas of

New York or London.[4] In addition, as I will argue throughout this book, the effects of relative poverty on the lives of children and their families are not insignificant and are at the root of many of the problems facing the so-called post-industrial nations. Social, health and economic policies which minimise or ignore 'first world poverty' have been pursued by governments which have enthusiastically supported economic stringency for debtor countries in the 'third world'; these policies can be shown to further exacerbate the problems of 'first' and 'third world' poverty (*see* Chapter 10).[13]

Child poverty in the USA

By 1995, almost 15 million US children under the age of 18 were living in families with incomes below the official poverty lines, and 6 million of these were under six years of age. Poor children make up 21% of US children under 18 and 24% under six.[14] Officially, 43.5% of black American children and 37.6% of Hispanic American children live in poverty.[15] On average, the incomes of their families fall short of the poverty lines by about US$4500, and a quarter of the families in poverty fall through all safety-net programmes and receive no form of government benefit.

Longitudinal data (Table 2.2) indicate that between 3 and 5 million US children live in persistent poverty, of whom the majority are black Americans. These children live in segregated neighbourhoods and the economic and social situation of their families as well as their reduced educational opportunities ensure that they remain in poverty.[15]

Child poverty in the USA showed a marked decline from 22.7% in 1964 to 14.2% in 1973. Poverty rates remained stable during the 1970s but underwent a sharp increase in the early 1980s to reach a high of 21.8% in 1983 (Figure 2.3). Subsequently, the level fell to 19% in 1988, rising again to 21.9% in 1992. Since 1992 there has been a slight decline in the proportion of poor children down to 21%.

An important trend in the USA, also noted in the UK and Europe (*see* below), is the increasing proportion of children amongst the poor.[15,16]

Table 2.2 Poverty and welfare receipt: 1985 levels and estimates of persistence. (Source [15] p. 26)

	All persons	*All children*	*Black children*
Persons (millions)			
1 Population totals	236.75	62.02	9.41
2 Official poor	33.06	12.48	4.06
3 Pre-welfare poor	35.17	13.02	4.23
4 AFDC* recipients	10.90	7.23	3.25
5 Persistently poor	11.57–20.83	2.98–4.71	2.72–3.20
6 Persistent AFDC recipients	5.92	2.98–4.05	1.96–2.54
Rates (percentages)			
Official poverty rate (rows 2/1)	14.0	20.1	43.2
Persistent poverty as a percentage of official poverty (rows 5/2)	35.0–63.0	23.9–37.7	67.0–78.8
Persistent poverty as a percentage of population (rows 5/1)	4.9–8.8	4.8–7.6	28.9–34.0
Percentage of pre-welfare poor receiving welfare (rows 4/3)	31.0	55.5	76.8
Percentage of persistently poor receiving welfare in a given year	57.0	69.6	n.a.
Percentage of official poor who are persistent welfare recipients (rows 6/2)	17.9	23.9–32.5	48.3–62.6
Percentage of population that is persistently welfare dependent (rows 6/1)	2.5	4.8–6.5	20.8–27.0

*AFDC = Aid to families with dependent children.

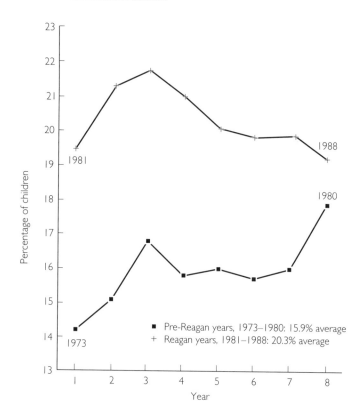

Figure 2.3   Trends in child poverty in the USA, 1973–88.
(Source [15])

Child poverty in the UK, the rest of Europe and other industrialised countries

Variations in official poverty measures and the absence of reliable figures for many countries make accurate estimates of the extent of child poverty problematic. Data are available for individual countries and comparisons of time trends are valid if within-country measures are constant. Table 2.3 shows time trends and figures for countries for which data are available.

More recent figures than those shown in Table 2.3 show that by 1992 the proportion of UK children in poverty had risen to 31%,[17] rising further to 34% in 1995–96.[18] Table 2.4 shows

Table 2.3 Trends in child poverty in selected countries.
(Source [16] p. 29)

	Around 1970	Around 1975	Around 1980	Around 1985
Canada	18.0	16.9	15.9	17.0
Czechoslovakia	–	11.4	9.3	8.2
Germany (FR)	14.0	7.4	8.7	8.9
Hungary	–	17.1	–	20.0
Ireland	–	15.7	18.5	26.0
Japan	–	25.3	12.8	10.9
Sweden	7.5	–	6.8	–
UK	–	–	9.0	18.1
USA	15.0	17.0	17.9	20.1

Table 2.4 Percentage of children in workless and poor
households, Europe. (Source [18] p. 66)

	In workless households (%)	In poor* households (%)
UK	19	32
Ireland	16	27
Portugal	3	26
Spain	10	25
Italy	7	24
Luxembourg	3	23
Greece	4	19
Netherlands	9	16
Belgium	11	15
Germany	4	13
France	9	12

*A poor household is one with an income below 50% of the median.

that the UK has the highest proportion of children living in
workless and poor households of all the EU countries. Based
on the 1991 Canadian census, the percentage of children aged
0–17 living in poverty remained at 17%, varying from 14% in
Prince Edward Island to 20% in Manitoba.[19] Between 1986 and

1995, the proportion of Australian children aged 0–15 years who were living in families in receipt of Additional Family Payments, a means-tested benefit, doubled from 20.1% to 40.6%.[20]

In many of the former socialist countries, the change to market economies has been accompanied by a dramatic increase in child poverty. The former Czechoslovakia (*see* Table 2.3) had shown a falling level of child poverty up to 1985, but child poverty has increased dramatically in the now Czech Republic, as it has in Poland and Romania.

As discussed in Chapter 1, differences in definition and measurement of poverty are considerable between countries. In the UK, the reluctance of successive governments to define official poverty lines has fuelled a major debate on definition and measurement (*see* Chapter 1, p. 5), one result of which has been experimentation with alternative approaches to poverty measurement (*see* p. 11). The UK child poverty figures in Table 2.3 are based on the official EU measure of less than 50% of the national mean household income. Using the consensus or subjective measures developed by Mack and Lansley, it is possible to estimate not just a child poverty figure, which was slightly higher than the EU measure for 1983, but also the numbers on the margins of poverty and in various degrees of poverty (Table 2.5).[21]

Despite the obvious limitations of the data, some tentative conclusions can be drawn. There has been a general upward trend in child poverty in developed countries, which accelerated in the late 1970s and early 1980s in line with the US experience. The upward trend appears to have been sharpest in the UK and Ireland; in a few countries, notably Japan and Sweden, the trend is reversed or the official child poverty levels have remained stable.

Not only has there been an increase in child poverty but there has been a trend for children to take over from the elderly as the group most likely to be in poverty. Table 2.6 compares trends in poverty among the elderly with those among children in three European countries.

This trend towards increasing poverty among children relative to the rest of the population is well illustrated in Figure 2.4,

Table 2.5 Number of children and adults in poverty as defined by a consensus view, Britain 1983–90. (Source [17])

Degree of poverty	Children 1983 Number (%)	Children 1990 Number (%)	Adults 1983 Number (%)	Adults 1990 Number (%)	Total 1983 Number (%)	Total 1990 Number (%)
In or on the margins	4.2	–	7.9	–	12.1	–
	–	–	–	–	(22.2)	–
In poverty	2.5	3	5.0	8	7.5	11
	–	–	–	–	(13.8)	–
Sinking deeper	1.4	–	3.3	–	4.7	6
	–	–	–	–	(8.6)	–
In intense poverty	0.9	–	1.7	–	2.6	3.5
	–	–	–	–	(4.8)	–

Table 2.6 Comparison of trends in child and elderly poverty in three European countries. (Source [16])

Country	Around 1970 (%)	Around 1975 (%)	Around 1980 (%)	Around 1985 (%)
Germany (FR)				
Elderly	11.9	9.0	8.6	6.5
Children	14.0	7.4	8.7	8.9
Ireland				
Elderly	–	34.8	25.0	10.0
Children	–	15.7	18.5	26.0
Sweden				
Elderly	9.0	–	1.5	–
Children	7.5	–	6.8	–

showing the increase in UK children living below 50% of average income level, after taking account of housing costs, compared with the rest of the population between 1979 and 1987.[22]

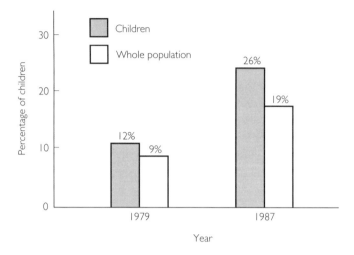

Figure 2.4   Trend in proportion of children compared with whole population living below 50% of national income level after housing costs in the UK, 1979 and 1987. (Source [22] p. 367)

Thus child poverty is increasing in many European countries and children are becoming the 'new poor'.

Factors underlying child poverty trends in developed countries (*see also* Appendix)

Factors contributing to the upward trend in child poverty vary from country to country. The following discussion is based primarily on UK and US data representing extreme examples of the trend; where available, contrasting data are presented from other countries.

Economic factors

These trends are associated with interrelated economic, social policy and demographic changes. The world economic recession, which began in the 1970s but had its most devastating effects on employment in the early 1980s, underpins these trends. In market economies, growth in gross domestic product

(GDP) per capita fell from an average of 4–5% in the 1950s and 1960s to 1–2% in the period between 1980 and 1989. The centrally planned economies of the former USSR and Eastern Europe also experienced a marked slow-down in growth.

Unemployment rates were relatively stable between 1949 and 1979 throughout the developed world: for example the US figure remained around 5%. In most developed countries unemployment rose steeply in the early 1980s, reaching a peak in 1983 of 9.5% in the USA and around 11% in the UK. Unemployment has disproportionately affected those under 30 and those in ethnic minorities. In addition, there have been marked regional differences in unemployment rates within countries. Average rates for the years 1983–86 in the UK varied from 7.9% in the south east to 16.2% in Northern Ireland. Within cities even more striking differences are evident, with unemployment rates for electoral wards varying between 3% and greater than 30% in a city-wide survey of unemployment carried out in Sheffield in 1985.[23]

Since the break-up of the former Soviet Union and the command economies of Eastern Europe there has been a massive increase in unemployment, particularly affecting Russia. Russia has experienced a tenfold increase in absolute poverty (those living on less than £2.40 per day) in the ten years since the dissolution of the Soviet Union.

Income changes

The general trend in the market economies towards an increase in earnings and spending power, noted throughout the 1950s and 1960s, suffered a major reverse as a consequence of the world recession. In the 20 years between 1949 and 1969 the incidence of low earnings in the USA declined rapidly from 40% to 11.8%; however, by 1986, despite a general increase in incomes, the level had risen again to 20.6%. In all years, black and Hispanic Americans had higher rates than white Americans, as did less educated men, but the least educated experienced the greatest deterioration in economic status up to 1986.[15] The percentage of US men who were earnings-poor increased from 12% of whites, 26% of Latinos and 32% of African-Americans in 1969 to 20%, 38% and 42%, respectively, in 1989. In the UK, the number of workers earning less than the Council of Europe's 'decency threshold', 68% of all full-time workers' mean earnings, rose from 7.8 million in 1979 to 10 million in 1991; ethnic minority groups, young workers and women are most likely to experience low pay.[17]

Income inequality increased sharply in the 1980s in a number of industrial market economies (Table 2.7).

In the USA, the inflation-adjusted income of the poorest quintile of families with children fell by 20% to US$7125, compared with a rise of 10% for the richest quintile to US$77 000.[24] The real disposable income of the poorest 5% of the UK population fell between 1979 and 1991 and families with children were most likely to have experienced an actual reduction in real income.[25,26]

Social policy in response to the slow-down in economic growth has varied between countries. The monetarist policies pursued, particularly in the USA and the UK, have aimed to reduce public expenditure and control money supply in order to combat inflation. Welfare programmes have suffered as a consequence; housing benefit, which supports the housing expenses of those on low incomes, and unemployment benefit, have been steadily eroded in the UK, and in the US the percentage of workers covered by unemployment insurance (UI) fell from 75% in 1975 to 31% in 1987 as a direct result of legislation restricting the scope of the UI programme.[15,17] With the possible exception of some Northern European countries, most family allowances have lagged behind in financial terms and have failed to adjust to the profound demographic changes discussed below.[16]

Table 2.7 Increase in income inequality. (Source [16])

	Year	Australia	UK	USA	Canada
Share of top 20%	1979–80	43.4	36.0	39.1	42.0*
	1985–87	45.4	42.0	41.7	43.2
Share of bottom 40%	1979–80	14.6	22.0	19.2	3.8
	1985–87	14.2	17.3	17.2	4.7

*refers to 1977.

The level of tax and credit transfers in different countries has a profound effect on low income rates in households with children and lone-parent households (*see* Chapter 10, Figures 10.2 and 10.3).[27] Comparison of the USA and Sweden is particularly striking: 17% of households with children and 40% of lone-parent households who would have been low income reduced to 2% and 3%, respectively, after tax and transfers in Sweden, compared with 25% and 68% reduced to only 22% and 56% in the USA.

The downward trend in poverty amongst the elderly and the parallel increasing trend amongst children, which seems to be happening in most developed countries (*see* above), is partly explained by a marked increase in government cash transfers to the elderly compared with children. In the USA, for example, in 1960 the ratio of elderly:children expenditure was 3:1, but by the late 1980s it had become 10:1.[28] This change represented both a reduction in welfare programmes for families with children and an increase in entitlements for the elderly.

Lone-parent families

Most industrial countries have experienced a rapid rise in lone-parent families (*see* Figure 2.5) as a result of the increased divorce rate and the increased tendency for children to be born outside marriage (*see* Table 2.8).

By 1986, 26% of US children under 18 were living in lone-parent families compared with less than 10% in 1960 – by far the greatest rate of increase in the developed countries (*see* Figure 2.5). In the UK, the number of dependent children living in lone-parent families increased from 1.45 million to 2.2 million in 1991.[17] Lone-parent households are mainly headed by women, with the result that approximately half the poor US children now live in households with a female head.[28] Lone-parent households are concentrated in inner-city areas and, especially in the USA, there is a disproportionate representation of ethnic minority children amongst them.

Lone parenthood is both a cause and a consequence of poverty. Between 1979 and 1990, the percentage of UK children in lone-parent families with incomes below half the

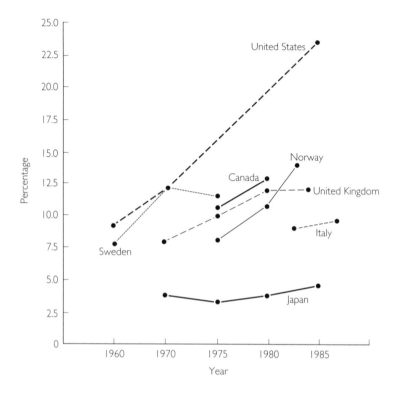

Figure 2.5 The rise in lone-parent families in various countries. (Source [16])

Table 2.8 Children born outside marriage. (Sources [15,17])

Country	% births outside marriage around				
	1950	*1960*	*1970*	*1980*	*1990*
UK	4	5	10	12.5	30
USA	4	5.3	10.7	18.4	22 (1985)
Sweden	–	–	–	42	–
Denmark	–	–	–	38*	–

*many of these births are to consensual unions rather than to single women.

average income increased from 28% to 74%.[17] There is evidence from the USA that economic and social policy changes, particularly long-term male unemployment, have played a role in generating these trends.[28] A study of teenage pregnancy and unemployment as part of the OPCS Longitudinal Study in the UK shows that unemployment precedes pregnancy, supporting the findings from qualitative research suggesting that motherhood is a 'career choice' for teenage girls living in areas with few job prospects.[29,30]

Summary

1   With a few notable exceptions, child poverty has increased in developed and less developed countries throughout the 1980s.

2   The world economic recession has adversely affected children in less developed countries by the massive drain of resources in debt repayments and in developed countries by the huge increase in unemployment.

3   The major demographic changes affecting family structure in developed countries, with a sharp increase in lone-parent families, has contributed to the increase in child poverty.

4   In less developed countries children remain the age group most vulnerable to poverty; in developed countries, children have displaced the elderly as the largest age group in poverty.

References

1   Haines A, Heath I and Smith R (2000) Joining together to combat poverty. *BMJ.* **320**:1–2.

2   Ebrahim GJ (1985) *Social and Community Paediatrics in Developing Countries.* Macmillan, London.

3   Navarro V (ed.) (1982) *Imperialism, Health and Medicine.* Pluto Press, London.

4   Townsend P (1993) *The International Analysis of Poverty.* Harvester Wheatsheaf, Hemel Hempstead.

5 Grant J (1994) *The State of the World's Children.* Oxford University Press, New York.

6 United Nations Development Programme (1994) *Human Development Report 1994.* UNDP & Oxford University Press, New York.

7 Sanders D (1985) *The Struggle for Health.* Macmillan Education, London.

8 Godlee F (1993) Third World debt. *BMJ.* 307:1369–70.

9 Save the Children Fund (1995) *Towards a Children's Agenda: New Challenges for Social Development.* Save the Children, London.

10 Unicef (1992) *Children of the Americas: Child Survival, Protection and Integrated Development in the 1990s.* Unicef Regional Office for Latin America and the Caribbean, Bogota, Colombia.

11 World Bank (1993) *World Development Report: Investing in Health.* Oxford University Press, New York.

12 Logie DE and Woodroffe J (1993) Structural adjustment: the wrong prescription for Africa? *BMJ.* 307:41–4.

13 Hewlett SA (1993) *Child Neglect in Rich Nations.* Unicef, New York.

14 Lewit EM, Terman DL and Behrman RE (1997) Children and poverty: analysis and recommendations. *Future of Children.* 7:4–24.

15 Danziger S and Stern J (1990) *The causes and consequences of child poverty in the United States.* Innocenti Occasional Papers, No. 10, Unicef International Child Development Centre, Florence, Italy.

16 Cornia GA (1990) *Child poverty and deprivation in industrialised countries: recent trends and policy options.* Innocenti Occasional Papers, No. 2, Unicef International Child Development Centre, Florence, Italy.

17 Kumar V (1993) *Poverty and Inequality in the UK: The Effects on Children*. National Children's Bureau, London.

18 NCH Action for Children (1999) *Factfile 2000*. NCH Action for Children, London.

19 Lochhead C and Shillington R (1996) *A Statistical Profile of Urban Poverty*. Center for International Statistics, Canadian Council on Social Development, Ottawa, Canada.

20 Birrell B, Maher C and Rapson V (1997) Welfare dependence in Australia. *People and Places (Center for Population and Urban Research, Monash University)*. **5**:68–77.

21 Mack J and Lansley S (1985) *Poor Britain*. George Allen and Unwin, London.

22 Spencer NJ and Graham H (1995) Children in poverty. In *Social Paediatrics* (eds B Lindstrom and NJ Spencer). Oxford University Press, Oxford.

23 Sheffield Health Authority (1991) *Health Care and Disease: A Profile of Sheffield*. Sheffield Health Authority, Sheffield.

24 US House of Representatives Committee on Ways and Means (1990) *Background Material and Data on Programs within the Jurisdiction of the Committee on Ways and Means*. US Government Printing Office, Washington DC.

25 University of Swansea Department of Economics (1994) *Winners and Losers*. Department of Economics, University of Swansea, Swansea.

26 Townsend P (1991) *The Poor are Poorer: A Statistical Report on Changes in Living Standards of Rich and Poor in the UK, 1979–89*. University of Bristol, Department of Social Policy and Social Planning, Bristol.

27 Ross D, Scott K and Kelly M (1996) *Child Poverty: What Are The Consequences?* Center for International Statistics, Canadian Council on Social Development, Ottawa, Canada.

28 Wise P and Meyers A (1988) Poverty and child health. *Pediatr. Clin. North Am.* **35**:1169–86.

29 Penhale B (1989) *Associations Between Unemployment and Fertility Among Young Women in the Early 1980s: Longitudinal Study Working Paper, No. 60.* OPCS, London.

30 Spencer NJ (1994) Teenage mothers. *Curr. Paediatr.* **4**:48–51.

3

Measuring child health

Introduction

The measurement of poverty was considered in Chapter 1. In this chapter, the equally important question of measuring child health is addressed. Health is difficult to define: it has been regarded as an absence of illness or, in the comprehensive World Health Organization (WHO) definition, as 'a state of complete physical, mental and social well-being and not merely the absence of disease or infirmity'.

Paradoxically, health status measures at all ages have been based on death: mortality rates have been the mainstay of comparisons between and within countries. Infant mortality rate (IMR) and under-five mortality rate (U-5MR) are recognised as measures not just of death rates in infancy and early childhood but also of the health and social status of whole populations.[1]

However, although mortality rates form the bulk of child health status data on which the study of the effects of poverty and low socio-economic status has been based, many other measures have been used and new measures are being developed. The impetus for this move to alternative child health status measures is the dramatic fall in mortality rates in developed countries since the beginning of this century (*see* Chapter 5) so that, beyond the first year of life, death has become a rare event.[2] There has been an increasing focus on measures of morbidity, growth and so-called 'positive' health measures. Measures of self-reported health and illness developed for use in adults have been adapted and developed for use with older children and adolescents, and measures of quality of life have been applied to children with specific medical conditions and to child populations.[3-8]

This chapter reviews the uses and limitations of various measures of child health, with particular reference to those which have been used to study the links between poverty and child health (*see* Chapters 4, 5 and 6). Mortality is considered first, followed by morbidity as medically defined and self-reported, growth and birthweight and other measures which are in various stages of development. The chapter concludes with an assessment of the value of different child health status measures in the study of the effects of poverty in various national and international settings.

Mortality

Mortality rates have been collected routinely in many developed countries since the 19th century (*see* Chapter 5) and in less developed countries since the early part of the 20th century (*see* Chapter 6). Inter- and intranational comparisons of health status continue to depend mainly on mortality data. For example, international monitoring of IMR and life expectancy has enabled the United Nations Development Programme (UNDP) (*see* also Chapter 6) to identify countries which are either ahead or behind the trend in health gains and, on a national level, the conclusions of the Black Report, which did much to reopen the debate on health inequalities in the UK, were based on Decennial Mortality Reports from the Registrar General's office.[9,10] Despite the fall in child mortality in developed countries, mortality rates are likely to remain the mainstay of health status measures, particularly in relation to international comparisons.

IMR and U-5MR are the most commonly published rates in childhood. IMR has been the traditional measure which reflects the general health status of the population and has been used in both developed and less developed countries. Unicef and the UNDP (*see* Chapter 6) have started to use the U-5MR more frequently as it better reflects the health experience of children in less developed countries. As Millard has argued, the focus on infant mortality may underestimate the adverse health experience of young children in less developed countries, as many are protected in their first year from the worst effects of undernutrition and unsafe water by prolonged breast-feeding.[11] Conversely, U-5MR may be inappropriate for comparing child health status within and between developed countries as death after the first year is so unusual that grouping these deaths together with infant deaths may lead to distortions of the data, owing to differences in population size.

Other early infancy and childhood mortality rates are less commonly used for international comparison but are published locally and nationally. The perinatal mortality rate (PMR) and the early and late neonatal mortality rates (ENMR and LNMR) are particularly useful in the study of pregnancy outcomes and the influence of service interventions and innovations such as neonatal intensive care. Post-neonatal mortality rate (PNMR), at least in developed countries, was thought to be a particularly sensitive measure of social difference in child health status. Although PNMR continues to show a marked social gradient (*see* Chapter 7), the numbers of deaths in this age group are now so small in some areas as a result of the decline in sudden infant death syndrome (SIDS) that its value as a health status indicator is questionable.[12]

In developed countries, deaths in later childhood suffer the same problem of diminishing numbers. Mortality rates at these ages, now dominated in developed countries by accidental deaths, are useful in large populations as indicators of differential injury exposure and experience. In late childhood and adolescence, mortality rates continue to reflect accidental deaths but also self-harm, and are useful indicators of trends in this important aspect of the mental health of young people.

Death rates by cause at various ages are particularly valuable in exploring social gradients in infant and child health outcomes. Respiratory, infectious and diarrhoeal deaths are particularly high in less developed countries (*see* Chapter 6). A similar pattern of infant and child mortality was seen in today's developed countries in the 19th century (*see* Chapter 5) and deaths from these causes continue to show a very marked social gradient in developed countries.[13,14] Accidental deaths show the same social gradient, with deaths due to house fires in the UK showing a particularly marked gradient.[13] Suicides in the 10–24 age group are also strongly socially related.[15]

Morbidity

Whilst morbidity measures overcome some of the problems of small numbers associated with mortality, measures based on ill health have their own inherent weaknesses and some which they share with death. Morbidity, like mortality, is a measure of illness and not of health. Clearly death is incompatible with any definition of health, but people can be 'healthy' despite having chronic diseases or disabling conditions. Definition and classification of morbidity is fraught with difficulties: ICD coding, even when adapted for paediatric use, focuses on rare pathologies and is inappropriate for the classification of many childhood illness episodes; disease classification is equally problematic, with definitional difficulties and problems of severity grading associated with even the most common childhood illnesses, such as asthma.[16,17]

Medically defined morbidity

Many of the available medically defined morbidity data are based on health service contacts. The majority of these are hospital contacts – either admissions or visits to hospital departments and specialist services. These are a rich source of illness data and have been used as health indicators in various studies and reports.[18–20] They can be analysed as all-cause or cause-specific contacts. In countries such as the UK, with a strong tradition of first-contact healthcare outside hospital, first-contact morbidity data provide a valuable data source.

Service contacts are influenced by a range of variables such as access, availability, differences in illness behaviour and, in some countries, financial barriers. As a consequence, morbidity data based on them are potentially unreliable. Hospital activity is known to vary greatly between and within countries, and diagnoses and treatment undergo change according to fashion.

The limitations of service contact data can be minimised in a number of ways: well-defined conditions, such as bacterial meningitis in childhood, which in developed countries are never knowingly managed at home, can be used as sentinel or marker conditions; for less well-defined conditions, such as childhood asthma and bronchiolitis, measures of severity can be judged on the basis of the level of nursing and medical intervention required.[21] However, these modified service contact measures are unlikely to be collected on a routine basis as they require careful case ascertainment and review of case records.

Dental caries in childhood is important both as a measure of morbidity and as an indicator of socio-economic differences.[22,23] In the UK regular dental health surveys are carried out in childhood, giving data on trends. Immunisation uptake is a good morbidity proxy: it is reasonable to assume that fully immunised children will not contract certain childhood infections and, conversely, individuals and child populations with inadequate immunisation uptake can be regarded as potentially unhealthy.[24] In developed countries, immunisation uptake is strongly influenced by social circumstances; in less developed countries, poor children are less likely to be immunised because of lack of access to health services.[24]

Self-reported morbidity

In order to overcome some of the limitations of morbidity data defined by service contact, measures of self-reported health and illness have been developed (*see* above). The development of these measures has been prompted partly by the assault on the medical model of health and illness which, *inter alia*, challenges the 'right' of doctors to define health and illness and argues that lay or patient definitions are equally valid.[25]

Self-reported data related to long-standing illness have been routinely collected as part of the General Household Survey in the UK and, for the first time in 1991, have formed part of the UK Census. More detailed self-reported data have been collected in an extensive UK Disability Survey.[26] Parent-reported morbidity data formed an important part of the longitudinal data collected in the three UK national cohort studies which have been a rich source of community-based morbidity data.[27]

A range of validated measures of self-reported health and illness are available that are suitable for adults (*see* above). Self-completed health status indicators have been developed for use in older childhood and adolescence. These focus on functional health and have been used mainly to study the health of children who have been treated for specific conditions such as leukaemia.[6] More extensive measures of quality of life in childhood have been developed.[8] A measure of parent-reported infant and child health and illness experience has been developed and tested in a large birth cohort.[28]

Self-reported morbidity measures have been criticised on the grounds that the same question can have different meanings for different social and cultural groups, rendering the responses invalid at least for comparing between group differences.[29] However, despite these reservations, a number of studies have demonstrated a marked negative social gradient for self-reported health and morbidity.[30–33] Further study of the problems of comparing self-reported health and illness across socially and culturally diverse groups is needed before these measures can be fully validated in the comparison of the health and illness experience of different social and cultural groups, but the social gradient, in the predicted direction which they consistently show, tends to legitimate their guarded use for this purpose.

Birth weight and growth

Birth weight is measured in many countries, less developed as well as developed. Although not a direct measure of health, the strong association of low birth weight (LBW) with adverse health outcomes in infancy makes it a good proxy measure of child health.[34] LBW rates are highly positively correlated with perinatal, neonatal and infant mortality rates. LBW is far more common than perinatal or infant death, so differences between regions and populations are more readily monitored and real changes over time can be better distinguished from random fluctuations.[35] The association of LBW rates with social and material deprivation makes it a particularly valuable measure of health inequalities between regions and child populations.[36]

Mean birth weight for whole populations or population subgroups is a valuable measure in assessing health status and has been shown to be valuable in exploring social differences.[36,37] Birth weight presented as means or as rates in 500 g bands provides additional information which can complement LBW rates alone. Wynn and Wynn have shown that the optimal birth weight for survival in developed countries lies between 3000 and 4500 g: banding allows between- and within-population comparisons of the percentages falling within this range as well as study of specific groups of special interest, such as very low birth weight (VLBW) babies (<1500 g).[38]

Various parameters of growth are measured frequently in infancy and childhood in both developed and less developed countries. Occipitofrontal circumference (head circumference) is measured at birth and during early childhood in some countries: its place as a screening procedure for the early detection of hydrocephalus has been debated but it has no place as a general measure of health in child populations. Weight measurement is widely used in developed and less developed countries to monitor early childhood growth and nutrition and as a screening procedure for failure to thrive (FTT).[39,40] In less developed countries, weight for height has been used to measure levels of undernutrition in child populations, but in developed countries weight monitoring has been questioned both as a health indicator and as a screening procedure for FTT.[21,41]

Height is the best recognised and most robust growth parameter in the study of the health of populations. Mean height has been shown to increase with increasing living standards and height trends provide vital historical data for studying the health and social experience of populations (*see* Chapter 4, p. 86).[42] Height seems to be a sensitive indicator of the nutritional and health status of populations and population groups even when differences related to different genetic pools are taken into account (*see* Chapters 6 and 8).[42,43] Routine measurement of height is problematic and open to error. However, simple measurement techniques are available that are applicable to developed and less developed countries and cross-sectional and longitudinal research studies can provide valuable population trends data.[44]

Other measures

Measures based on the 'new morbidity', such as behavioural problems and rates of child abuse and neglect, are increasingly important in view of the rise in prevalence of these health-related problems in developed countries.[45] Behavioural measures have been proposed as part of child surveillance programmes.[46] Psychiatric morbidity measures are increasingly important in older childhood and adolescence in developed countries.[47]

Jolly suggests a range of measures in the study of the effects of poverty on child health. She states:

> *In assessing health it is useful to consider both physical and psychosocial markers of health. It is also useful to assess not only health deficits, i.e. morbidity and mortality, but also the preceding events, i.e. the absence of the positive health marker that led to the presence of the marker of a health deficit before continuing to the health deficit itself. For example, the absence of the health marker 'adequate antenatal care' is associated with increasing prevalence of markers of health deficits in this population, e.g. maternal anaemia. This in turn is associated with a worse obstetric outcome which is the health deficit itself.* ([48] p. 39)

Table 3.1 shows Jolly's novel approach to health and health deficit markers at the extremes of childhood.

The danger in Jolly's approach is that some of the measures she suggests are themselves SES measures, such as 'safe and pleasant environment', and others, for example lack of school readiness and poor school performance, although health-related, are measures of educational attainment and not health. However, immunisation and breast-feeding levels, which she describes as positive health markers, are widely accepted as

Table 3.1   Health and health deficit markers associated with poverty or low SES at the extremes of childhood. (Source [48])

A Age group: 0–4		
	Physical	Social/psychological
Absence of a positive health marker	• normal length gestation • normal birth weight • breast-fed • immunisation complete • well child care received	• adequate care • adequate interaction between mother and child • continuity of healthcare • safe and pleasant environment • access to services
Presence of a health deficit marker	• prematurity • low birth weight • poor nutrition • elevated lead level • iron-deficiency anaemia	• developmental delay
Presence of a disease or disability	• stillbirth rate increased • perinatal mortality rate increased • infant mortality – 1 mth–1 yr increased • SIDS • mortality 1–4 yrs • injury • suboptimal growth • otitis media/hearing loss • respiratory infections • gastroenteritis • hospitalisation rates • child abuse	• lower than expected IQ • behaviour disorders

continued overleaf

Table 3.1   Continued

B Age group: 15–18		
	Physical	Social/psychological
Absence of a positive health marker	• adequate dental care	• adequate school progress • access to services • adequate self-esteem • knowledge about contraception/STDs
Presence of a health deficit marker	• substance abuse • pregnancy	• lower self-esteem
Presence of a disease or disability	• increased mortality • injury • hepatitis B carrier prevalence • poor dental status	• school failure • suicide and attempted suicide • delinquency

health proxies in that their absence is strongly correlated with negative health outcomes in the way Jolly suggests in the quotation.

Child health measures in the study of health inequalities

As will be seen in Part Two (Chapters 4, 5 and 6), there has been a multitude of studies showing the relationship between child health and poverty and low SES, and a variety of different measures have been used. My purpose here is to summarise my view of the child health measures which are particularly suited to exploring the relationship, not to give a comprehensive list of all the measures which could be or have been used. Where appropriate, the limitations of particular health measures are considered in the text in the following chapters, where the detailed evidence is considered as well as in Part Three (Chapters 7, 8 and 9), which is concerned with causal explanations and interpretations.

Mortality

Death rates remain the mainstay of child health status measures internationally and are particularly useful in the comparison of large child populations. The following rates are valuable in studying health inequalities:

- IMR – SIDS deaths in developed countries; respiratory and gastrointestinal infection deaths in both developed and less developed countries

- U-5MR – respiratory and gastrointestinal infection deaths in less developed countries; accidental deaths, particularly fire deaths, in all countries

- 5–9MR – accidental deaths in all countries

- 10–14MR – accidental deaths in all countries; suicides and self-harm deaths in developed countries and countries in rapid developmental transition

- 15–18MR – accidental deaths in all countries; suicide deaths.

Morbidity

Medically defined

- hospital admission rates for marker conditions such as bacterial meningitis and accidents

- dental caries using standardised measure

- psychosocial morbidity – parasuicide in older children; behavioural problems in younger children in developed countries

- primary care contact rates for marker conditions.

Self-reported

These require further work but are widely used to study long-standing illness.

Birth weight and growth

- LBW rates

- mean birth weight

- birth weights by 500 g bands

- percentage of births outside optimal range (3000–4500 g)

- mean heights attained at different ages

- weight for height in less developed countries.

Other measures

These are measures which are not strictly measures of ill health or positive health but are either proxies or health deficit markers:[48]

- breast-feeding rates – especially in less developed countries where the relationship between artificial feeding and ill health in infancy is strong

- immunisation uptake.

References

1   Grant J (1994) *The State of the World's Children.* Oxford University Press, New York.

2   Kohler L (1991) Infant mortality – the Swedish experience. *Annu. Rev. Public Health.* 12:177–93.

3   Hunt SM, McKenna SP, McEwan J *et al.* (1980) A quantitative approach to perceived health status: a validation study. *J. Epidemiol. Community Health.* 34:281–6.

4   Brazier JE, Harper R, Jones NMB *et al.* (1992) Validating the SF-36: a new outcome measure for primary care. *BMJ.* **305**:160–4.

5   Starfield B, Bergner M, Ensminger M *et al.* (1993) Adolescent health status measurement: development of the Child Health and Illness Profile. *Pediatrics.* **91**:430–5.

6   Barr RD, Furlong W, Dawson S *et al.* (1993) An assessment of global health status in survivors of acute lymphoblastic leukaemia in childhood. *Am. J. Pediatr. Hematol. Oncol.* **15**:284–90.

7   Rosser R, Cottee M, Rabin R *et al.* (1992) Index of health-related quality of life. In *Measure of Quality of Life* (ed. A Hopkins). Royal College of Physicians of London, London.

8   Lindstrom B (1995) Measuring and improving quality of life for children. In *Social Paediatrics* (eds B Lindstrom and NJ Spencer). Oxford University Press, Oxford.

9   United Nations Development Programme (1994) *Human Development Report 1994*. UNDP and Oxford University Press, New York.

10   Townsend P and Davidson N (1982) *Inequalities in Health: The Black Report*. Penguin, Harmondsworth.

11   Millard AV (1994) A causal model of high rates of child mortality. *Soc. Sci. Med.* **38**:253–68.

12   Gilbert R (1995) New developments in SIDS: the case of the 'back-to-sleep' campaign. In *Progress in Community Child Health* (ed. NJ Spencer). Churchill Livingstone, Edinburgh.

13   Woodroffe C, Glickman M, Barker M *et al.* (1993) *Children, Teenagers and Health: The Key Data*. Open University Press, Milton Keynes.

14   Danziger S and Stern J (1990) *The causes and consequences of child poverty in the United States*. Innocenti Occasional Papers, No. 10, Unicef International Child Development Centre, Florence, Italy.

15 Gunnell DJ, Peters TJ, Kammerling RM *et al.* (1995) Relation between parasuicide, suicide psychiatric admissions and socioeconomic deprivation. *BMJ.* **311**:226–30.

16 British Paediatric Association (1987) *British Paediatric Association Classification of Diseases* (2e). BPA, London.

17 Hoskyns EW, Heaton DM and Beardsmore CS (1991) Asthma severity at night during recovery from an acute asthma attack. *Arch. Dis. Child.* **66**:1204–8.

18 Spencer NJ and Lewis MA (1991) Multiple admissions under 2 years of age. *Arch. Dis. Child.* **66**:938–40.

19 Hill A (1989) Trends in paediatric medical admissions. *BMJ.* **298**:1479–82.

20 Northern Territory Health (1986) *Health Indicators in the Northern Territory.* Northern Territory Health Department, Darwin, Australia.

21 Spencer NJ, Logan S, Scholey S *et al.* (1996) Deprivation and bronchiolitis. *Arch. Dis. Child.* **74**:50–2.

22 Prendergast MJ, Beal JF and Williams SA (1993) An investigation of non-response bias by comparison of dental health in 5-year-old children according to parental response to a questionnaire. *Community Dent. Health.* **10**:225–34.

23 Carmichael CL, Rugg-Gun AJ and Ferrell RS (1989) The relationship between fluoridation, social class and caries experience in 5-year-old children in Newcastle and Northumberland. *Br. Dent. J.* **167**:57–61.

24 Logan S and Bedford H (1995) Implementing immunization programmes. In *Social Paediatrics* (eds B Lindstrom and NJ Spencer). Oxford University Press, Oxford.

25 Capewell S (1994) Are health and illness defined by society or by doctors? *Proc. Roy. Coll. Physicians Edinburgh.* **24**:181–6.

26   Bone M and Meltzer H (1989) *The Prevalence of Disability Among Children. OPCS Survey of Disability in Great Britain: Report 3*. HMSO, London.

27   Golding J (1984) Britain's National Cohort Studies. In *Progress in Child Health, Vol. 1* (ed. JA Macfarlane), Churchill Livingstone, Edinburgh.

28   Spencer NJ and Coe C (1996) The development and validation of a measure of parent-reported child health and morbidity: the Warwick Child Health and Morbidity Profile. *Child Care.* **22**:367–79.

29   Blane D, Power C and Bartley M (1996) Illness behaviour and the measurement of class differentials in morbidity. *J. Roy. Stat. Soc.* **Series A. 159**:77–92.

30   Power C, Manor O and Fox J (1991) *Health and Class: The Early Years*. Chapman and Hall, London.

31   Arber S (1987) Social class, non-employment and chronic illness: continuing the inequalities in health debate. *BMJ.* **294**:1069–74.

32   Children's Defense Fund (1992) *The Health of America's Children, 1992: Maternal and Child Health Data Book*. Children's Defense Fund, Washington DC.

33   Brannen J, Dodd K, Oakley A *et al.* (1994) *Young People, Health and Family Life*. Open University Press, Milton Keynes.

34   Macfarlane A and Chalmers I (1981) Problems in the interpretation of perinatal mortality statistics. In *Recent Advances in Paediatrics, No. 6* (ed. D Hull). Churchill Livingstone, Edinburgh.

35   Logan S (1991) Outcome measures in child health. *Arch. Dis. Child.* **66**:745–8.

36   Elmen H (1995) *Child Health in a Swedish City: Mortality and Birth Weight as Indicators of Health and Social*

Inequality. The Nordic School of Public Health, Goteborg, Sweden.

37 Spencer NJ, Bambang S, Logan S *et al.* (1999) Socio-economic status and birth weight: comparison of an area-based measure with the Registrar General's social class. *J. Epidemiol. Community Health*. 53:495–8.

38 Wynn A and Wynn M (1981) *The Prevention of Handicap of Early Pregnancy Origin*. Foundation for Education and Research in Child-Rearing, London.

39 Wright C (1995) A population approach to weight monitoring and failure to thrive. In *Recent Advances in Paediatrics, No. 13*. (ed. T David). Churchill Livingstone, Edinburgh.

40 Ebrahim GJ (1985) *Social and Community Paediatrics in Developing Countries*. Macmillan, London.

41 Hall DMB (1991) *Health for All Children* (2e). Oxford University Press, Oxford.

42 Tanner JM (1989) *Fetus into Man* (2e). Castlemead Publications, Ware, Herts.

43 Martorell R (1984) Genetics, environment and growth: issues in the assessment of nutritional status. In *Genetic Factors in Nutrition* (eds A Velasquez and H Bourges). Academic Press, New York.

44 Carr-Hill R (1995) Trends in childhood mortality and morbidity. In *Social Paediatrics* (eds B Lindstrom and NJ Spencer). Oxford University Press, Oxford.

45 Haggarty R, Roghmann K and Pless I B (1975) *Child Health in the Community*. Wiley, New York.

46 Stoddart P (1995) New thought on the management of behavioural problems in preschool children. In *Progress in Community Health* (ed. NJ Spencer). Churchill Livingstone, Edinburgh.

47 Rutter M and Smith D (eds) (1995) *Psychological Disorders in Young People*. Wiley, Chichester.

48 Jolly DL (1990) *The Impact of Adversity on Child Health: Poverty and Disadvantage*. Australian College of Paediatrics, Parkville, Victoria.

Part Two

Evidence of child health inequalities

4

Historical evidence linking poverty and child health in developed countries

Introduction

This chapter explores historical evidence related to child health inequalities in countries which have experienced dramatic improvements in health and life expectancy during the last 100 years in order to inform the current debate on the effects of poverty on child health. The chapter, along with the others in this section, seeks to establish the continuities and links between the determinants of child health in developed countries before the beginning of the 20th century and those in the less developed (Chapter 5) and developed countries (Chapter 6) of today.

Historical data are necessarily limited. With some notable exceptions, which are considered below, very few studies highlighting child health inequalities were undertaken at the time. However, descriptive evidence is available and retrospective research has been carried out on routinely collected data and other data sources. I start by exploring available mortality and morbidity data for evidence of child health inequalities before going on to compare child health indicators for pre-20th century Europe with those of present-day less developed countries. The final part of the chapter explores the determinants of the fall in infant mortality and the rise in life expectancy which occurred in developed countries over the last 100 years.

Child health inequalities

Between-country differences

As with the less developed countries of today, there is some evidence of marked differences in infant and child mortality between countries in Europe in the 18th and 19th centuries and differences in the speed and pattern of change over time (*see* below). In Vienna, Austria, in the 1750s, the IMR was reported to be 410/1000 whereas the figure for Sweden during the same period was given as 203/1000.[1] The IMR for France for the ten-year period 1790–99 was 255/1000, for Sweden during the same period it was 210/1000 and for England approximately 170/1000.[2,3] Later in the 19th and early 20th centuries, clear differences are evident between countries, as shown in Table 4.1.

It is also interesting to note that the steady decline in infant mortality which occurred from 1920 onwards is not reflected in these figures. They show considerable year-on-year variation for each country, although Sweden does demonstrate a steadier rate of decline than the others. This is further demonstrated in Figure 4.1, which shows the fall in IMR indexed by three-year moving means, with each country's 1891 IMR taken as 100.

These mortality differences are related to socio-economic factors and levels of development but, as can be seen in the discussion of the determinants of the mortality decline in Europe (*see* below), although socio-economic factors had an important role, there were other key variables which modified their effects to different degrees in different settings.

In an interesting study which explores the determinants of the improvements in life expectancy in Japan from 1900 to 1960, Johansson and Mosk compare the Japanese experience with that of England and Wales and Italy, both more industrially developed than Japan at the turn of the 20th century.[4] Figure 4.2 shows the pattern of life expectancy in the three countries between 1900 and 1980.

The important point to note is the similarity in life expectancy early in the 20th century between the three countries

Table 4.1 Variations in IMR among selected European countries, 1881–1913. (Source [6])

Year	England and Wales	Scotland	France	Belgium	Netherlands	Sweden	Prussia	Italy
1881	130	112	165	155	182	113	199	–
1882	141	118	165	151	175	125	208	–
1883	137	119	165	154	187	116	211	–
1884	147	118	177	168	194	113	213	–
1885	138	120	162	150	169	114	204	–
1886	149	116	173	178	192	111	225	–
1887	145	122	161	145	162	103	199	–
1888	136	113	165	165	173	100	198	–
1889	144	121	155	160	177	107	207	–
1890	151	131	176	166	171	103	210	192
1891	149	128	161	162	169	108	201	188
1892	148	117	181	169	174	109	211	184
1893	159	136	173	165	164	101	206	180
1894	137	117	158	152	152	101	196	184
1895	161	133	180	172	167	95	212	187
1896	148	115	148	142	148	103	191	177
1897	156	138	152	149	148	99	205	165
1898	160	134	169	160	156	91	193	169
1899	163	131	163	167	149	112	204	156

continued overleaf

Table 4.1 Continued

Year	England and Wales	Scotland	France	Belgium	Netherlands	Sweden	Prussia	Italy
1900	154	128	161	172	155	99	212	172
1901	151	129	142	142	149	103	200	165
1902	133	113	135	144	130	86	172	175
1903	132	118	137	155	135	93	194	168
1904	145	123	144	152	137	84	185	164
1905	128	116	136	146	131	88	198	166
1906	132	115	143	153	127	81	177	160
1907	118	110	135	132	112	77	168	155
1908	120	121	129	147	125	85	173	153
1909	109	108	120	137	99	72	164	155
1910	105	108	111	134	108	75	157	142
1911	130	112	117	167	137	72	188	153
1912	95	105	78	120	87	–	146	130
1913	108	110	–	–	91	–	–	–

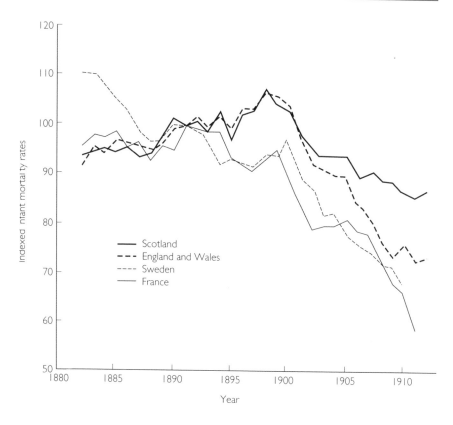

Figure 4.1 Indexed three-year moving means of infant mortality rates (1891 = 100) for Scotland, England and Wales, Sweden and France 1882–1912. (Source [6])

despite the marked differences in per capita income shown in Table 4.2.

Johansson and Mosk postulate that the Japanese 'high achievement' in life expectancy despite its low per capita income was due to the highly effective public health measures and level of literacy existing in Japan at that time. The plateauing of life expectancy from 1910 onwards and the sharp fall during the Second World War appear to have been related to the initial effects of urbanisation on public health measures and the direct effects of war. Johansson and Mosk comment:

> *The mortality history of Japan is unique in many ways. One point, which has not been widely appreciated, is*

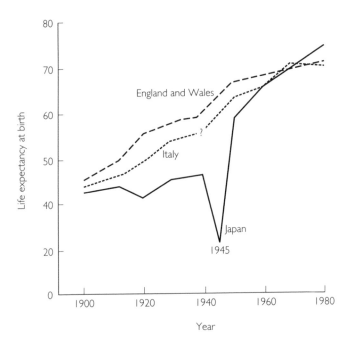

Figure 4.2   Life expectancy at birth (males), 1900–80, Japan, Italy and England and Wales. (Source [4])

> *that Japan was the first country to use its cultural and political institutions to demonstrate what is observed in Costa Rica, Kerala State, China and several other areas today – above a certain fairly minimum standard of living threshold, the 'right' to live to old age can be secured for the average citizen, even in low-income developing countries, if the government is dedicated to the efficient exploitation of existing public health technology and the population is educated and cooperative.* ([4] p. 235)

The high achievers amongst the less developed countries are considered in more detail in Chapter 5. The Japanese experience serves to show the importance of public health measures in the decline in mortality (*see* below).

Table 4.2 Income, mortality and mediating variables – comparison of Japan, Italy and England and Wales in 1900. (Source [4] p. 217)

	Resistance proxies[a]		Exposure proxies[b]		Protection from exposure		Mortality variables		
	Income per head (1963 US$)	Adult height, males (cm)	Urban (%)	Primary industry (%)	Public health type	Education, per cent literate	e_0 (M)	e_{10} (M)	IMR (M + F)
Japan (1908)	68 (100*)	157	10	70	National and very efficient	90	43	49	155
Italy (1901)	226 (300*)	163	14	60	National and moderately efficient	30	43	51	174
England/ Wales (1901)	551 (550*)	169	54	15	Local and inefficient	95	45	50	154

[a] proxies for factors which are thought to protect against mortality
[b] proxies for factors which entail exposure to increased risk of mortality
* income figure adjusted for non-market sector of the economy

Regional (within-country) differences

Data are available from British counties in 1861 which demonstrate considerable regional differences in IMR.[5] Lancashire had the highest IMR of 174/1000, with the East Riding of Yorkshire second highest with a rate of 171/1000, whereas Grampian and the Highlands in Scotland both had rates of 86/1000. Lee interprets these differences as indicating that the majority of high IMR counties were the industrialising counties of the English midlands and north.[5] In his analysis of trends in regional differences between 1861 and 1971, he shows that the national decline in IMR was not evenly reflected throughout the regions and that the two most powerful explanatory variables for high levels of IMR over time were levels of industrial, particularly mining, employment and the ratio of high- and low-density living accommodation.

Both the regional variation and the changing pattern over time (1861–1990) can be seen in Figure 4.3.

Comparisons between IMRs for cities over time are also interesting. The IMRs show considerable fluctuations as well as clear differences between cities and rural areas (*see* Figure 4.4).

In 1870 the IMR for Liverpool was more than twice that of North Devon and considerably higher than Birmingham and London. Despite fluctuations, the differential between Liverpool and North Devon remained fairly constant throughout the 40 years from 1870 to 1910. London showed a fall in IMR after 1890, whereas Birmingham showed an increase which brought it up to a similar rate to Liverpool by the early 1900s. Woods and co-workers explain the fall in London rates and the continued high rates in Liverpool as follows:

> *In many middle-class areas or suburban districts (of London) there was little or no increase in infant mortality during the 1890s, but their share of London's population increased. In the inner of East End districts infant mortality did increase but the effect on London as a whole was dampened. Liverpool was in some ways similar to London's East End, mortality*

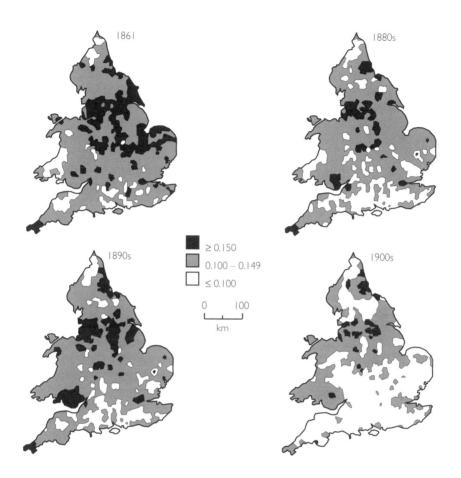

Figure 4.3 Variations in infant mortality for England and Wales, 1861, 1880s, 1890s and 1900s. (Source [6])

was exceptionally high and increased somewhat during the 1890s, but in the outer districts of Liverpool (West Derby and Toxteth Park) the Birmingham pattern was followed more closely. ([6] p. 360)

Differences between socio-economic groups

The Great Plague of London in 1665 was one of the first occasions on which systematic recording of deaths, in the form

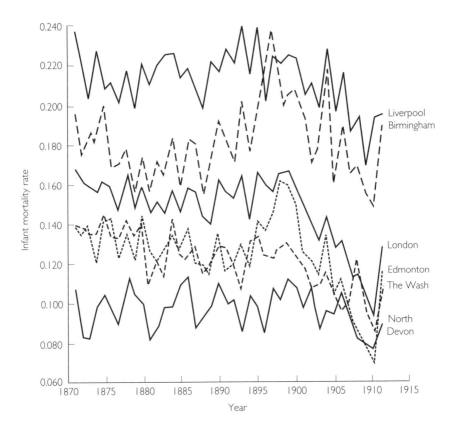

Figure 4.4   Infant mortality time series for selected English cities and rural areas, 1871–1911. (Note: Liverpool, Birmingham and Edmonton are single registration districts. London is a registration division. The Wash and North Devon are combinations of six registration districts.) (Source [6])

of the Bills of Mortality, permitted the relationship between poverty and disease to be noted. Defoe wrote of that period:

> *The misery of that time lay upon the poor, who, being infected, had neither food nor physic, neither physician nor apothecary to assist them.*[7]

In fact, it seems that malnutrition, overcrowded living conditions and the inability to flee infected areas, rather than the attentions of physicians, were the factors which determined the higher mortality among the poor. The weekly Bills of Mortality were used by the more prosperous residents as an early warning to flee the area.[8] Even before the Great Plague devastated London, plague had been endemic and intermittently epidemic in the British Isles since its entry into the country in 1348. Howe states that:

> Rattus rattus *(the carrier of the plague bacillus) found conditions congenial in the lowly dwelling houses crowded together in 14th-century towns. Stone-built houses of the well-to-do were not so congenial to them. Thus bubonic plague was primarily and principally a disease of the poor.* ([9] pp. 114–15)

The pioneers of the public health movement, Villerme in France and Chadwick in England, were among the first to draw attention to the relationship between low social class and mortality and morbidity.[10,11] In the 1820s Villerme used the connection between mortality and untaxed rents in Paris to examine mortality differentials between social groups. Annual rents of more than 150 francs were taxed; those below 150 francs were untaxed and were seen as an indicator of poverty. Villerme grouped each district of Paris (*arrondissement*) according to the percentage of untaxed rents and noted a positive correlation between high percentage untaxed rents and deaths per 1000 inhabitants (Table 4.3).

Chadwick showed similar differences in his 'Report on the Sanitary Conditions of the Labouring Population of Great Britain' published in 1842.[11] The report of an 1844 Royal Commission compares percentages of children under five years dying in the families of different occupational groups in the town of Preston in the North West of England: 17.6% of the children of the gentry died before the age of five years compared with 55.4% of the children of labourers, weavers and factory hands. Expressed as under-five mortality rate (U-5MR) – often used in less developed countries in addition to IMR (*see* below and Chapter 6) – the children of the gentry had an U-5MR of 176/1000 and the children of labourers etc. had an U-5MR of 554/1000.[12]

Table 4.3   Average annual mortality for rich and poor in Paris as indicated by the taxation level of each *arrondissement*, 1817–21. (Source [8] p. 214)

Arrondissement	Untaxed rents (%)	Deaths per 1000 inhabitants
2	7	16.1
3	11	16.7
1	11	17.2
4	15	17.2
11	19	19.6
6	21	18.5
5	22	18.9
7	22	19.2
10	23	20.0
9	51	22.7
8	32	23.3
12	38	23.3

An insight into the reasons for this carnage among the children of the poor can be gained from the following extract, originally published in the *Health of Towns Magazine and Journal of Medical Jurisprudence* of 1847–48, which describes living conditions in poor tenement buildings in Westminster, London:

> *On entering these houses you have a fine specimen of the manner in which the lower orders of Westminster live. Living by day and night in one wretched room, with scarcely any light – an intermittent supply of water, and a shocking fetid atmosphere – full of rags and filth – it is dreadful! In the corner of the room may be seen what may be termed an apology for a bed and bedding, being a mass of rags piled together, in the midst of which are the poor sickly children, whose very countenances bespeak that they will soon cease to trouble their parents; with hair uncombed, barefooted and in rags – with their skin unwashed – the majority of them never live to manhood, while*

one third die before they attain the age of five years. The adult inhabitants, also, have all the appearance of being always in a typhoid state. The courts and alleys in this colony of filth and fever are chiefly un-paved and undrained, and mostly with but one privy for one court, which contains, sometimes upwards of twenty houses ... Such is a brief sketch of a portion of what is commonly known as Lower Westminster, and which is situated midway between Buckingham Palace and the House of Lords and Commons, and about 300 yards from either.[12]

A recent study based on the analysis and linkage of primary data sources for the northern English city of Sheffield for the period 1870–71 demonstrates a marked seasonal variation of infant mortality for the whole city, with more deaths in the period July to September, related to the higher number of deaths associated with diarrhoea in the warm summer months.[13] Williams shows the influence of both environment and social class on a seasonal infant mortality index constructed so that if there were no seasonal differences the index for each season would be 100 (Figure 4.5).

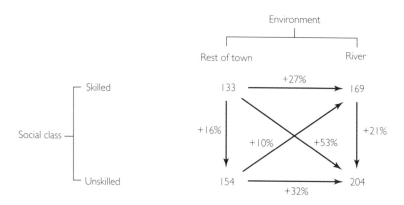

Figure 4.5   Infant mortality: seasonal infant mortality index values for Sheffield, July–September 1870–71, by environment and social class. (Source [13])

This figure shows marked differences in seasonal mortality between the infants of skilled and unskilled workers in whichever part of the city they lived, but the most vulnerable were infants of unskilled workers living in the low-lying river areas of the city.

Other evidence for the health differential between social groups in 19th-century Europe comes from a study of the records of the Rotunda Maternity Hospital in Dublin, Ireland, between 1801 and 1840.[14] From the records, the percentage of children reported alive of those ever-born was calculated and the percentages for wealthy and poorer districts compared. In 1824, 64.9% of the ever-born children were reported alive in wealthy districts compared with 60.3% in the poorest districts. Kass reports that the European royal families had an IMR of 12/1000 towards the end of the 19th century, which contrasts sharply with IMRs for European countries during the same period.[15]

Moving forward to the early part of the 20th century, data from a number of US and European sources show striking differences in IMRs for children in different income groups.[1] These are summarised in Table 4.4.

The IMR ratios between low and high income groups are consistently more than 2:1, and for post-neonatal mortality rate (PNMR) the ratios exceed 5:1.

The above discussion has focused on IMRs as data have been routinely collected in many countries for many years. Another powerful indicator of health for which data are available from the 19th and the early part of the 20th century is height.

Tanner[16] maintains that the tradition of growth studies and the science of auxological epidemiology grew out of the reactions of humanitarians to the appalling conditions of the poor and their children.

Villerme, one of the earliest auxological epidemiologists, in 1829 observed marked regional differences in height among young men in France, concluding as follows:

Human height becomes greater and growth takes place more rapidly, other things being equal, in proportion

Table 4.4a Infant, neonatal and post-neonatal mortality rated by earnings of father, seven American cities, 1912–15. (Source [1])

Father's annual income	Mortality rates			Mortality ratios		
	Infant	Neonatal	Post-neonatal	Infant	Neonatal	Post-neonatal
$1250 or more	59	38	21	100	100	100
$1050–1249	64	33	31	108	87	148
$850–1049	83	38	45	141	100	214
$650–849	108	46	62	183	121	295
$550–649	117	43	74	198	113	352
$450–549	126	46	80	214	121	381
Less than $450	167	56	111	283	147	529
No earnings	211	61	150	358	161	714
Not reported	140	41	99	237	108	471
Total	110	44	66	186	116	314

Father's annual income per capita						
$400 or more	60			100		
$200–399	96			160		
$100–199	123			205		
$50–99	142			237		
Less than $50	216			360		
Total	110			183		

Table 4.4b Stillbirth, infant, neonatal and post-neonatal mortality rates and ratios by family income, Stockholm, 1919–22. (Source [1])

Annual income	Mortality rates			
	Stillbirths	Infant	Neonatal	Post-neonatal
10 000 Kr. or more	9	14	11	3
6000–9999 Kr.	13	32	20	12
4000–5999 Kr.	16	38	15	23
Less than 4000 Kr.	18	49	24	25
Total	–	37	18	19
	Mortality ratios			
10 000 Kr. or more	100	100	100	100
6000–9999 Kr.	148	223	173	421
4000–5999 Kr.	180	268	132	800
Less than 4000 Kr.	199	341	211	855
Total	–	264	164	633

Table 4.4c Infant, neonatal and post-neonatal mortality rates and ratios by median rented census tract grouping, whites only, Cleveland five city area, 1919–37. (Source [1])

Economic tenth	Mortality rates				Mortality ratios			
	1919–23	1924–28	1929–33	1934–37	1919–23	1924–28	1929–33	1934–37
				Infant mortality				
Highest	42	37	33	32	100	100	100	100
2	50	48	42	38	118	128	130	117
3	50	46	44	37	119	123	133	115
4	51	48	44	36	121	128	136	118
5	61	54	47	38	144	146	143	116
6	64	57	51	38	151	153	157	116
7	64	56	52	40	153	149	160	123
8	73	65	58	47	173	173	178	144
9	81	69	56	53	192	184	171	163
Lowest	104	86	66	48	246	229	203	150
Total	73	60	50	41	173	160	154	126
				Neonatal mortality				
Highest	30	28	24	26	100	100	100	100
2	36	33	30	29	120	119	129	113
3	32	33	31	25	108	119	133	98
4	34	34	31	26	112	122	133	100
5	36	34	32	26	122	125	137	99

Table 4.4c Continued

Economic tenth	Mortality rates				Mortality ratios			
	1919–23	1924–28	1929–33	1934–37	1919–23	1924–28	1929–33	1934–37
6	37	35	32	28	124	126	136	106
7	35	34	33	27	115	124	142	105
8	38	36	36	31	125	131	154	121
9	39	35	32	32	129	126	136	123
Lowest	41	39	34	29	136	142	144	110
Total	37	35	32	28	123	126	136	107
Post-neonatal mortality								
Highest	12	10	9	6	100	100	100	100
2	14	15	12	8	112	156	133	134
3	18	13	12	12	146	137	134	189
4	18	14	13	10	145	145	143	163
5	24	20	14	12	199	204	159	189
6	27	22	19	10	220	227	213	161
7	30	22	19	12	247	221	208	198
8	35	28	22	15	293	291	242	245
9	42	34	24	21	349	351	264	332
Lowest	63	46	32	20	520	473	356	323
Total	36	25	18	13	297	256	203	206

as the country is richer, comfort more general, houses, clothes and nourishment better and labour, fatigue and privation during infancy and youth less; in other words, the circumstances which accompany poverty delay the age at which complete stature is reached and stunt adult height. ([16] p. 162)

According to Tanner,[16] (p. 163), Villerme's explanation was challenged by Boudin, an army surgeon, who maintained that the differences were due to altitude, climate and race. This debate in early 19th-century France has interesting resonance for the debate in less developed countries (Chapter 5) and developed countries (Chapter 6) related to the determinants of height. It is an early example of the causal debate related to health inequalities (Chapter 8).

Figure 4.6 shows the trends in the heights of US-born white males from 1710 to 1930. The fluctuations challenge the commonly held view that there was a straightforward 'secular trend' in height which saw heights increasing steadily across generations.[17] Fogel, among others, has argued that these fluctuations represent the sensitivity of average height measures to changing living standards.[18] Similar fluctuations are

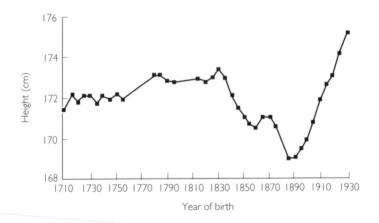

Figure 4.6   Trends in the heights of US-born white males, 1710–1930. (Source [18])

reported by Floud and co-workers in a study of British military recruits between 1740 and 1840, and they concluded that:

The early part of the industrial revolution led to an absolute as well as relative increase in the welfare and nutritional status of the working class but ... the impact of urban growth eroded this increase and even led to decreases in average height as large proportions of the working class were subjected to town life. ([19] p. 326).

Floud *et al.* also showed marked socio-economic inequalities in height: at the end of the 19th century they report that 13-year-old boys from the most privileged backgrounds were, on average, nearly 10 inches taller than their peers in the slums.[19] French army conscript data for 1868 show variation in height attained by occupational status and an income proxy.[20] The authors also report a close association of the height of the conscripts and their level of literacy, and conclude 'it is standard of living rather than way of life which produces this contrast in physical anthropology'.

The meticulous recording for commercial purposes of birth weights and heights of African slaves transported to and working in the USA and the Caribbean has enabled an extensive study of their birth weight, infant mortality and growth patterns.[21,22] The average birth weight was calculated as approximately 2.3 kg and their IMR 330/1000. The mean heights of US slaves are shown in Table 4.5.

The data indicate that the children of slaves were poorly nourished, but nourishment improved in both boys and girls when they reached working age and were able to command a larger share of resources. These data have also been used to illustrate the potential for 'catch-up growth' in adolescence, even in individuals whose growth has been stunted for long periods.[23]

As discussed in the previous chapter, birth weight, like height, is an indicator of health which can be used to study social groups within countries. Unlike height, historical sources of birth weight are rare; however, data from a Viennese maternity

Table 4.5 The mean height of US slaves compared with modern height standards. (Source [18])

Age (yrs)	Males			Females		
	Number	Height (cm)	Centile of modern standard	Number	Height (cm)	Centile of modern standard
1.5	96	60.7	0.0	91	60.1	0.0
2.5	136	74.1	0.0	148	74.9	0.1
3.5	187	84.7	0.2	168	82.9	0.1
4.5	195	91.2	0.3	206	91.2	0.5
5.5	169	97.2	0.3	200	99.0	1.6
6.5	218	103.2	0.5	262	101.6	0.4
7.5	200	110.8	1.5	241	110.0	1.8
8.5	281	114.6	0.9	337	115.5	2.2
9.5	266	121.0	1.7	306	119.6	1.4
10.5	557	125.1	1.6	528	124.6	1.4
11.5	347	131.9	3.6	443	130.4	2.1
12.5	751	135.2	2.4	736	134.8	0.9
13.5	470	141.1	3.0	556	142.0	0.9
14.5	732	146.6	2.1	765	148.0	1.7
15.5	571	153.0	1.3	812	152.4	5.6
16.5	709	158.1	1.2	1113	155.5	13.3
17.5	655	163.2	4.6	871	157.4	21.5
18.5	1142	165.7	8.9	1268	158.0	24.5
19.5	900	167.7	14.5	594	158.6	27.4
20.5	1527	168.5	17.6	1264	158.4	26.8
21.5	944	170.5	26.1	337	158.8	28.4
22.5	1374	170.2	24.8	664	159.0	29.5
23.5	795	170.6	26.8	404	158.8	28.4
24.5	872	169.9	23.6	442	159.4	31.9
25–49	8725	170.6	26.8	6552	159.8	34.5

hospital between 1865 and 1930 demonstrate, within the lower social groups, a clear social gradient in the proportion born low birth weight (<2500 g), from 13.6% among unemployed women to 7.5% among those employed in domestic service.[24]

Comparison of 19th- and early 20th-century USA and Europe with less developed countries today

Age patterns of mortality

The age pattern of deaths in less developed countries is different from that in present-day developed countries with the burden of mortality falling in the early years of life (*see* also Chapter 5). Eighteenth and 19th-century Europe had IMRs and U-5MRs of the same magnitude or higher than present-day less developed countries. This would suggest a similar age pattern of mortality. There is some fascinating evidence from 16th-century London based on parish records in the parish of St Botolph without Aldgate which, though not allowing calculation of mortality rates because of the absence of denominator data, can be used to look at the proportional mortality.[25] Figure 4.7 compares the proportional mortality of St Botolph

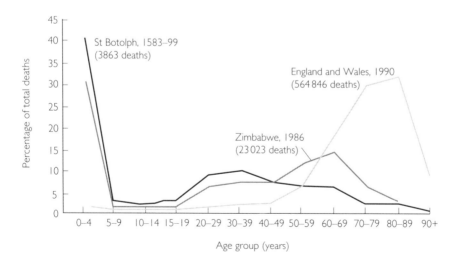

Figure 4.7 Proportional mortality by age group: St Botolph without Aldgate, 1583–99 compared with England and Wales, 1990 and Zimbabwe, 1986. (Source [25])

without Aldgate with that for Zimbabwe in 1986 and England and Wales in 1990.

The striking similarity of the proportional mortality for St Botolph without Aldgate and Zimbabwe suggests that factors threatening early childhood survival may have been similar in 16th-century London and 20th-century Zimbabwe; factors which are no longer present to the same degree in present-day London.

Pertussis (whooping cough) remains an important cause of death in less developed countries and affects mainly infants less than one year old. Infants are the most vulnerable to the condition. In present-day developed countries, pertussis still exists despite vaccination but tends to affect older children, at which time it is less dangerous. However, evidence from Aberdeen in Scotland at the end of the 19th century suggests that the age distribution of deaths from whooping cough was the same as it is in present-day less developed countries (*see* Figure 4.8).[12]

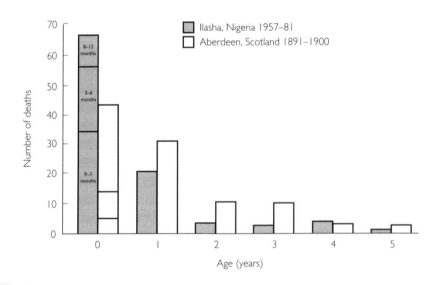

Figure 4.8   Age distribution of deaths from whooping cough: comparison of Aberdeen, Scotland, 1891–1900 and Ilasha, Nigeria, 1957–81. (Source [12])

Causes of death and ill health

Comparison of causes of death and ill health among children in pre-20th-century Europe and present-day less developed countries provides further evidence for the similarity between the health and illness experience of children in these different geographical and historical settings.

Sanders classifies most disease in less developed countries into two groups: nutritional and communicable – airborne and water-related and faecally transmitted (Table 4.6).[12]

Undernutrition (*see* above and Chapter 5) has a dual role as both a cause and an exacerbating factor of ill health. All the common infections of childhood are more likely to occur in undernourished children and are more likely to be severe.[12]

With few exceptions, the same diseases listed in Table 4.6 were responsible for high mortality and morbidity rates among children and adults in pre-20th-century Europe. Table 4.7 contrasts the death rates per million in England and Wales in 1848–54 and 1971 from a similar list of conditions to that depicted in Table 4.6.

In England and Wales in the 1860s, 6000 per million children under the age of 15 years died from scarlet fever, diphtheria, whooping cough and measles.[12] Tuberculosis (TB) death rates were equally high: in 1840, the rates were 4/1000. Summer diarrhoea was a major cause of death in childhood, as demonstrated by the work of Williams considered above, and Figure 4.9 shows how dysentery and diarrhoea in those over five years have diminished in importance since the mid-1800s.[13]

The so-called 'tropical diseases', often depicted as diseases of tropical physical and geographical conditions affecting only certain ethnic groups, were prevalent in Europe in the 19th century and some, such as TB, have never quite disappeared and are undergoing a revival.[9] Thus, these conditions can be seen as more socio-economic and environmental than tropical. Typhus, TB, cholera and many others were endemic in pre-20th-century Europe and were diseases of the poor, related directly to overcrowded and unhygienic living conditions and undernutrition.[9]

Table 4.6 Classification of most diseases in underdeveloped countries. (Source [12] p. 20)

Nutritional	Communicable		
	Airborne		Water-related and faecally transmitted
Undernutrition and associated vitamin deficiencies	Viral	Influenza Pneumonia Measles Chickenpox	Water-borne or water-washed: Cholera, typhoid, diarrhoeas, dysenteries, amoebiasis, infectious hepatitis, poliomyelitis, intestinal worms
	Bacterial	Whooping cough Diphtheria Meningitis Tuberculosis	Water-washed: Skin and eye infection Trachoma Skin infection Leprosy Scabies
			Skin infestation Louse-borne typhus
			Water-based: Penetrating skin Ingested Schistosomiasis (bilharzia) Guinea worm
			Water-related insect vectors: Biting near water Breeding in water Sleeping sickness Malaria Yellow fever Onchocerciasis (river blindness)

Key: airborne = disease spread by breathing airborne, respiratory secretions of infected persons; water-borne = disease transmitted when pathogen is in water which is then drunk by person who may then become infected; water-washed = disease whose prevalence will fall when increased *quantities* of water are used for drinking and hygienic purposes (the water should be clean, but need not be pure); water-based = disease where pathogen spends a part of its life cycle in an intermediate aquatic host or hosts.

Table 4.7   Death rates (per million) in England and Wales – comparison of 1848–54 with 1971. (Source [12] p. 30)

	1848–54	1971	% of reduction attributable to each category
Conditions attributable to micro-organisms (communicable):			
Airborne diseases	7259	619	40
Water- and food-borne diseases	3562	35	21
Other conditions	2144	60	13
Total	12 965	714	74
Conditions not attributable to micro-organisms:	8891	4070	26
All diseases	21 856	5384	100

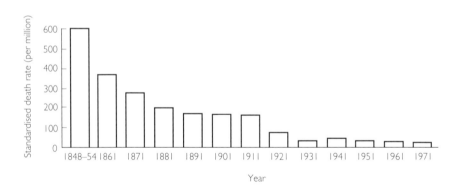

Figure 4.9   Decline in death rates at age five years and over from diarrhoea and dysentery, England and Wales, 1848–1971. (Source [12])

Further confirmation of this characterisation is the fact that populations living in very close geographical proximity, such as the white and black populations of South Africa, have very different disease patterns owing more to social and environmental than geographical or ethnic conditions.[8]

Explanations for the fall in mortality in developed countries during the 20th century

Medical developments and innovations are commonly thought to have been major determinants of the fall in mortality to the present levels which has taken place over the last 100 years in developed countries. In fact, as Figure 4.10 demonstrates, medical innovations, with a few notable exceptions such as smallpox vaccination, essentially came too late to influence the fall.

McKeown was among the first to challenge the medical view. He produced evidence to show the influence of economic growth, improved standards of living and improved nutritional standards on the fall in mortality. McKeown concentrated on TB, the single most important cause of death in the mid-19th century.[26]

McKeown's conclusions have been challenged on a number of grounds. Winter argues that McKeown concentrates too much on the biomedical role of medicine and ignores the potential educative role of doctors, for example in simple hygiene measures, and the role of what he calls 'indirect medical interventions'.[27] Others have criticised McKeown's failure to acknowledge the importance of medical interventions and knowledge related to smallpox and the influence of immunisation for conditions such as measles on morbidity rather than mortality.

The most consistent and convincing critique of McKeown is made by the social historian, Szreter.[28] Szreter does not dispute McKeown's conclusion that modern scientific medicine had little role in mortality decline. However, he does dispute McKeown's conclusion that rising living standards and nutrition were the main determinants of the decline. Szreter points out that TB, though the most important cause of death, was only one of a number of airborne diseases prevalent in the 19th century and was not typical. For many of these diseases, the decline could not be attributed to nutritional improvements alone: smallpox declined in response to vaccination; pneumonia and influenza

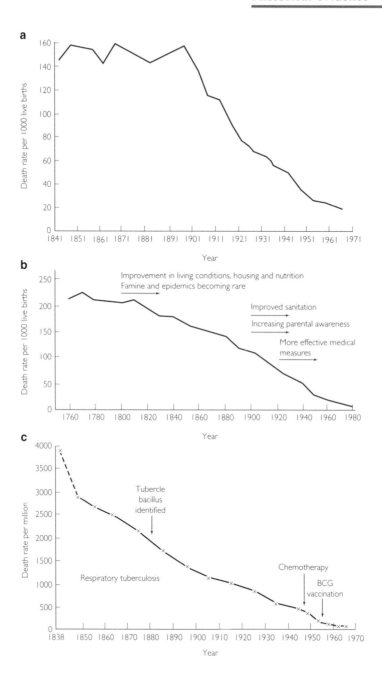

Figure 4.10 (**a**) IMR, England and Wales, 1841–1971; (**b**) social development and IMR in Sweden, 1760–1980; (**c**) death rate decline from respiratory tuberculosis, England and Wales, 1838–1970. (Sources [3,8])

actually increased as causes of death in the second half of the 19th century. Szreter focuses instead on the water- and food-borne diseases which declined in response to improved public health measures. He argues that economic growth itself does not guarantee health improvements: in fact, rapid urbanisation and consequent overcrowding may result in deterioration in health for those living in urban areas. Szreter stresses the importance of public health measures in the decline in mortality as well as the issue of distribution of the benefits of economic growth, which if distributed widely across the population will lead to health gains.

Szreter's analysis is supported by the evidence of Woods and co-workers, Lee, Johansson and Mosk, and Harris, which is considered above.[4–6,18,29] The fluctuations in mortality and in heights attained during the later part of the 19th century support the view that economic growth *per se* is no guarantee of health gain.

The lessons of Japan indicate that public health measures can greatly influence national health outcomes.

Summary

1   Inequalities in child health were present in pre-20th century Europe and USA.

2   Children living in poverty and poor economic circumstances in pre-20th century Europe and USA had poorer health outcomes than their more privileged peers.

3   Inter- and intra-country differences in infant and early childhood mortality in developed countries during the 19th century and the early part of the 20th century broadly reflected economic differences as well as differences in public health measures.

4   There are striking similarities between the patterns of child mortality in today's less developed countries and the patterns that existed in developed countries before the dramatic mortality decline.

5   'Tropical disease' is a misnomer: with very few exceptions, the major 'killer diseases' of the less developed countries today were those of the developed countries in the 19th century.

6   The decline in mortality in developed countries in the 20th century cannot be explained by medical advances but owes much to public health measures as well as more equitable distribution of the benefits of economic growth.

References

1   Antonovsky A and Bernstein J (1977) Social class and infant mortality. *Soc. Sci. Med.* **11**:453–70.

2   Woods RI (1993) On the historical relationship between infant and adult mortality. *Popul. Stud.* **47**:195–219.

3   Ebrahim GJ (1985) *Social and Community Paediatrics in Developing Countries.* Macmillan, London.

4   Johansson SR and Mosk C (1987) Exposure, resistance and life expectancy: disease and death during the economic development of Japan, 1900–1960. *Popul. Stud.* **41**:207–35.

5   Lee CH (1991) Regional inequalities in infant mortality in Britain, 1861–1971: patterns and hypotheses. *Popul. Stud.* **45**:55–65.

6   Woods RI, Watterson PA and Woodward JH (1988) The causes of rapid infant mortality decline in England and Wales, 1861–1921, Part I. *Popul. Stud.* **42**:343–66.

7   Defoe D (1966) *A Journal of the Plague Year.* Penguin, Harmondsworth.

8   Susser MW, Watson W and Hopper K (1985) *Sociology in Medicine.* Oxford University Press, New York.

9   Howe GM (1976) *Man, Environment and Disease in Britain: A Medical Geography Through the Ages.* Penguin, Harmondsworth.

10   Villerme LR (1826) Rapport fait par M. Villerme, et lu a l'Académie de Médicine, au nom de la Commission de Statistique, sur une série de tableaux rélatifs au mouvement de la population dans les douze arrondissements municipaux de la ville de Paris pendant les cinq années 1817–21. *Archives Générales de Médicine.* **10**:216–45.

11   Flinn MW (ed.) (1965) *Report on the Sanitary Conditions of the Labouring Population of Great Britain, by Edwin Chadwick, 1842.* Edinburgh University Press, Edinburgh.

12   Sanders D (1985) *The Struggle for Health.* Macmillan, London.

13   Williams N (1992) Death in its season: class, environment and the mortality of infants in nineteenth-century Sheffield. *Soc. Hist. Med.* **5**:71–94.

14   O'Grady C (1991) Dublin's demography in the early nineteenth century: evidence from the Rotunda. *Popul. Stud.* **45**:43–54.

15   Kass EH (1980) *Maternal Infection and Fetal Growth Retardation.* Paper presented at Unicef Conference, Boston, MA.

16   Tanner JM (1981) *A History of the Study of Human Growth.* Cambridge University Press, Cambridge.

17   Fogel R (1986) Nutrition and the decline in mortality since 1700: some preliminary findings. In *Long-term Factors in American Economic Growth* (eds S Engerman and R Gallman). University of Chicago Press, Chicago.

18   Harris B (1994) Health, height and history: an overview of recent developments in anthropometric history. *Soc. Hist. Med.* **7**:297–320.

19   Floud R, Wachter K and Gregory A (1990) *Height, Health and History: Nutritional Status in the United Kingdom, 1750–1980.* Cambridge University Press, Cambridge.

20   Ladurie EL and Bernageau N (1971) Étude sur un contingent militaire (1868): mobilité géographique, délinquance

et stature, mise en rapport avec autres aspects de la situation des conscrits. *Annales de Démographie Historique.* **xx**:311–17.

21   Steckel R (1986) A peculiar population: the nutrition, health and mortality of American slaves from childhood to maturity. *J. Econ. Hist.* **44**:721–41.

22   Steckel R (1986) A dreadful childhood: the excess mortality of American slaves. *Soc. Sci. Hist.* **10**:427–65.

23   Steckel R (1987) Growth, depression and recovery: the remarkable case of the American slaves. *Ann. Hum. Biol.* **14**:111–32.

24   Ward PW (1988) Birth weight and standards of living in Vienna, 1865–1930. *J. Interdiscipl. Hist.* **xix(2)**:203–29.

25   Gray A (ed.) (1993) *World Health and Disease.* Open University Press, Milton Keynes.

26   McKeown T (1976) *The Role of Medicine: Dream, Mirage or Nemesis?* The Nuffield Hospitals Trust, London.

27   Winter JM (1982) The decline in mortality in Britain, 1870–1950. In *Population and Society in Britain, 1850–1950* (eds T Barker and M Drake). Batsford Academic and Educational, London.

28   Szreter S (1988) The importance of social intervention in Britain's mortality decline, c. 1850–1914: a reinterpretation of the role of public health. *Soc. Hist. Med.* **1**:1–37.

29   Woods RI, Watterson PA and Woodward JH (1989) The causes of rapid infant mortality decline in England and Wales, 1861–1921, Part II. *Popul. Stud.* **43**:113–32.

5

Poverty and child health in less developed countries

Introduction

An estimated 250 million children live in poverty, over 90% of whom live in the less developed countries of the world (*see* also Chapter 2).[1] This chapter is concerned with the evidence for the influence of poverty on the health of children in less developed countries. Together with Chapters 4 and 6, it seeks to establish the continuity of the effects of poverty on the health of children over time and across different countries.

The literature related to poverty and child health in less developed countries is vast; it is not my intention to make an exhaustive review but to focus on evidence linking the economic and developmental status of countries with the health status of their populations and the evidence for child health inequalities within less developed countries. The chapter starts by contrasting the child health status of developed and less developed countries and examining the association between macroeconomic indicators, such as gross national product (GNP) and child health status measures. This is followed by more detailed examination of less developed countries, with particular emphasis on the countries which achieve good health status indicators despite low GNPs and those that have relatively poor health status indicators despite relatively high GNPs. Possible explanations for the differences in child health outcomes are explored briefly – they are addressed again in Part Three (The causal debate) and Part Four (Social and health policy implications).

Global comparisons of measures of child health status

International comparisons of health status measures can be presented in numerous ways. For the purposes of this book, the focus is on socio-economic variables and poverty levels and the evidence linking these to adverse child health outcomes. As considered in Chapter 1, GNP is a crude measure of national income but only very broadly reflects individual income and poverty levels within countries. The Human Development Index (HDI), developed by the UN Development Programme (UNDP), is the best index developed so far which takes account of income distribution within countries and other variables related to SES, such as female literacy.[2] In its disaggregated form (*see* below) it provides an even more powerful tool for regional and national comparison.

At the extremes of the developed and less developed worlds, the relationship between GNP and child health indicators is clear and strong. Table 5.1 contrasts child health status indicators for the ten countries with the lowest GNP per capita with those for the ten with the highest GNP per capita.

The poorest countries in terms of per capita GNP all show far higher levels of adverse child health outcomes than the richest. At this crude level, the relationship between the wealth of a country and the health status of its children is beyond dispute. When considered in terms of country groupings by under-five mortality rates (U-5MRs), the same strength of relationship is evident (Table 5.2).

Despite the clarity of the overall relationship of GNP to child health status of countries, some low GNP per capita countries achieve relatively good measures of child health status and in some high GNP per capita countries child health outcomes are relatively poor (*see* below for specific examples). It was in order to account for these important exceptions that the UNDP developed the HDI. It is important to note here that a component of the index itself is life expectancy, and child mortality rates bear a direct relationship to this component.

Table 5.1   Comparison of infant and child health indicators for ten high and ten low GNP per capita countries. (Source [3])

	IMR (1996)	U-5MR (1996)	Life expectancy at birth (1996)	% low birth weight (1990–94)
Low GNP per capita countries (US$100–180):				
Mozambique	133	214	47	20
Malawi	137	217	41	20
Chad	92	149	47	–
Somalia	125	211	48	16
Burundi	106	176	46	–
Nepal	82	116	56	–
Bangladesh	83	112	57	50
Tanzania	99	144	51	14
Laos	102	128	53	18
Rwanda	105	170	36	17
High GNP per capita countries (US$19 380–40 630):				
Japan	4	6	80	7
Sweden	4	4	78	5
Finland	4	4	76	4
Switzerland	5	5	79	5
France	5	6	79	5
Canada	6	7	79	6
Norway	5	6	77	4
Germany	5	6	76	6
Denmark	6	6	75	6
USA	8	8	76	7

Caution must be employed when interpreting the relationship between child health status measures based on mortality and HDI.

Table 5.3 shows weighted values for IMR and the percentage of underweight children aged less than five years for

Table 5.2   Health and other indicators by countries grouped according to U-5MR. (Source [4])

Indicator	Very high U-5MR countries* (>140)	Middle U-5MR countries (21–70)	Low U-5MR countries (≤20)
U-5MR	193	36	11
GNP per capita	US$295	US$1725	US$12 575
Life expectancy	49	70	76
Adult literacy	23%	86%	92%
Low birth weight (<2.5 kg)	17%	8%	6%
% household expenditure on food	53%	35%	12%
% access to safe water	44% (22% rural)	83% (64% rural)	100%

* High U-5MR countries (70–140) omitted to simplify the table.

Table 5.3   Trends in IMR and percentage of underweight children < five years in less developed countries by level of human development (HDI rank). (Source [2])

	IMR (per 1000 live births)		Underweight children (% of children <5)	
	1960	1992	1960	1992
High HDI countries (rank 20–52)	83	30	14	10
Medium HDI countries (rank 53–118)	139	40	29	22
Low HDI countries (rank 119–173)	165	98	57	48

developing countries, ranked by HDI and grouped into high, medium and low HDI countries.

Even between less developed countries there is a marked gradient in adverse child health outcomes, which is strongly associated with socio-economic factors, including national income and levels of adult literacy. Against a background of falling IMRs in most countries of the world, the trend in IMR and percentage of underweight children in the years between 1970 and 1992 is as expected with overall improvement. However, low HDI countries show a slower rate of reduction in both parameters. There is also evidence that if countries improve their HDI they tend to show a more rapid reduction in adverse child health outcomes.[2]

Detailed comparisons of less developed countries

I have considered above the limitations of GNP as a measure of income within countries and the need for a more comprehensive measure, such as HDI, which better explains national differences in child health outcomes. Figure 5.1 illustrates further the discrepancy between GNP and HDI despite the broad correlation.

This figure clearly illustrates the wide variation in HDI between countries with the same GNP per capita. Sri Lanka and China have per capita GNPs on a par with the Central African Republic but their HDIs are considerably better. Similarly, Hungary has a similar per capita GNP to South Africa and Algeria but performs much better in terms of HDI. Brief case studies of countries performing better and worse than expected for GNP help to illustrate some of the reasons for the differences. They also throw light on the socio-economic factors which influence child health outcomes in less developed countries.

Sri Lanka

Despite its low per capita GNP, Sri Lanka has adopted a national policy of more equitable income distribution linked

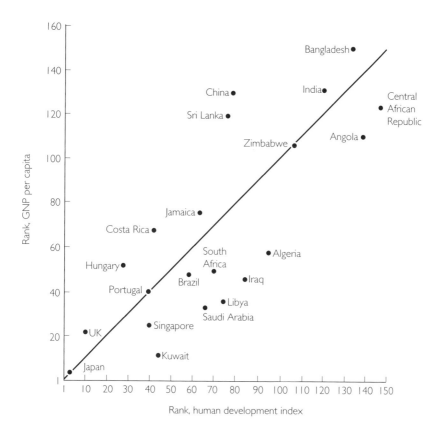

Figure 5.1 Relationship between GNP rank and HDI rank for selected countries (1992 data). Rank ordering: best = 1; worst = 160. (Source [2] p. 88)

with a system of food distribution based on ration books and coupons for essential commodities. This system includes food subsidies for low-income families and special protein-enriched food supplements for schoolchildren. More equitable income distribution means that when the HDI is adjusted for income distribution, Sri Lanka improves its rank in the 'HDI tables' by seven positions.[2]

In terms of child health outcomes, in 1996 Sri Lanka had an IMR of 17 and an U-5MR of 19. Table 5.4 compares the health outcomes and trends between 1960 and 1996 of Sri Lanka and

Table 5.4 Comparison of trends in IMR and U-5MR 1960–96 for Sri Lanka and Lesotho with similar GNP per capita in 1996. (Source [3])

	IMR		*U-5MR*	
	1960	*1996*	*1960*	*1996*
Sri Lanka (GNP per capita US$700)	90	17	130	19
Lesotho (GNP per capita US$520)	137	96	203	139

Lesotho, both of which had a GNP per capita of US$700 in 1996. The table shows the rapid improvements in both IMR and U-5MR of Sri Lanka compared with Lesotho.

China

Like Sri Lanka, China has had a long-standing policy of egalitarian income distribution. As a consequence, despite its low GNP per capita it has consistently achieved well in terms of human development. China has the largest positive gap between its HDI rank and its GNP per capita rank – +49 – in other words, when ranked in terms of HDI it rises 49 positions compared with its GNP per capita rank. Despite this remarkable achievement, there are still very marked regional differences in HDI related to the different income and adult literacy levels of the regions (*see* Figure 5.2).

As with Sri Lanka, China has shown rapid improvement in child health indicators: the IMR has fallen from 140 in 1960 to 38 in 1996, and the U-5MR in the same period has fallen from 209 to 47.[3]

These achievements in China may be in jeopardy as a result of the sharp increase in income inequality associated with the rapid shift to a market economy. China's Gini coefficient, a measure of income inequality (*see* Chapter 2), increased from 0.229 in 1988 to 0.307 in 1995.[5] Child health status measures do not yet reflect this shift but a deterioration, or at least a slowed rate of progress, is likely to occur as a result. Sharply contrasted to the mainland China experience is that of Taiwan where economic growth has been associated with a reduction in income inequality, which has been shown to have a highly significant effect on U-5MR.[6]

Kerala State

Though not a nation, Kerala State is an important example of a poor state within a large country which has achieved reductions in adverse child health outcomes by the use of state measures to redistribute income and increase adult literacy. (*See* Chapter 10, p. 285 for a more detailed discussion of the Kerala experience.)

Brazil

Brazil has not had a government policy of income redistribution or of increasing adult literacy. Between 1960 and 1983, the share of national income taken by the poorest 50% of the population fell from 17% to 13%, whereas that of the wealthiest 1% rose from 12% to 18%. Though the average GNP per capita of Brazil increased during the period, income distribution became more unequal. Brazil's GNP per capita rank is almost 20 positions higher than its HDI rank. Though sharply contrasted in terms of income redistribution policies, Brazil shares with China (and other countries) very marked regional differences in HDI, closely related to regional income (*see* Figures 5.2 and 5.3).

Despite having a GNP per capita almost six times that of Sri Lanka, in 1996 Brazil had an IMR of 44 and U-5MR of 52, both almost three times greater than Sri Lankan rates.[3] During the period 1960–82, when Brazil experienced an average annual growth rate of GNP per capita of 6.3%, the average annual reduction in U-5MR was 3.3% compared with an average reduction in U-5MR of 4.6% in Sri Lanka, which experienced a much slower GNP per capita average annual growth of 2.8%.

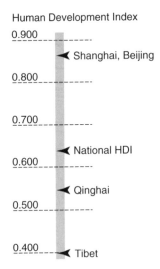

Figure 5.2   Human Development Index in China: national and regional HDIs. (Source [2] p. 101)

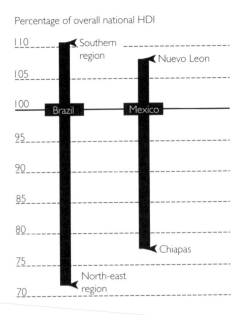

Figure 5.3   Regional HDI disparities in Brazil and Mexico. (Source [2] p. 99)

South Africa

South Africa is a particularly interesting though atypical example as a result of the apartheid policies practised by the National Party governments until recently. South Africa has a GNP per capita of US$2470, putting it among the upper middle income group of countries. However, its HDI rank is considerably lower as a result of the very different experiences of different ethnic groups within the country. Figure 5.4 shows life expectancy, GDP per capita expressed in PPP$ (Purchasing Power Parity – *see* Chapter 1) and HDI for white and black South Africans.

Child health outcomes for the different ethnic groups reflect these inequalities in HDI: in 1985, the IMR for white South Africans was 12.3/1000 compared with 51.9/1000 for 'coloureds' and 109/1000 for black South Africans.

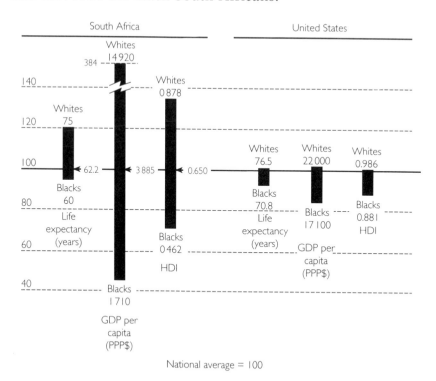

Figure 5.4 Disparities between HDIs for blacks and whites in South Africa and the United States. (Source [2] p. 98)

These case studies show that national income alone does not guarantee improved child health outcomes. Though income is a key determinant, levels of adult literacy, particularly female literacy, and income distribution play an important role in child health.

Child health inequalities in less developed countries

Child health experience is uneven in less developed countries just as it was (Chapter 4) and is (Chapter 6) in developed countries. Here, I concentrate on evidence for child health inequalities related to income and other socio-economically related factors such as maternal education. I will touch on the causes of these inequalities in the final section of this chapter, though Part Three focuses on causal mechanisms and the causal debate.

Regional variations

There is strong and consistent evidence for within-country regional differences in child health outcomes, as touched on above. Life expectancy is lower and infant mortality higher in the poorer areas of less developed countries: in China, life expectancy is lower in Tibet than in Shanghai; in Nigeria, life expectancy is 39.6 years in the region of Borno compared with 59.5 years in Bendel.[2] Data from Kenya in 1979 are shown in Figure 5.5.[1] This shows the difference in under-two mortality rate (U-2MR) between six rural provinces by the proportion of families below the poverty line in each province. The figure further illustrates the importance of maternal education and its protective effect in child health (*see* below for fuller discussion of the relationship between maternal education and poverty).

Childhood mortality in Southern Sudan is approximately 66% higher than in the north.[7] North-east Brazil, the poorest area of the country, has an infant mortality rate of 142/1000 live births compared with 44/1000 in the more affluent south.[8]

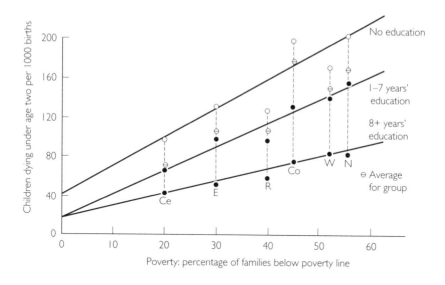

Figure 5.5 Child mortality by level of poverty and maternal education in six rural provinces of Kenya in 1984. Ce = Central, E = Eastern, R = Rift Valley, Co = Coast, W = Western, N = Nyanza. (Source [1])

Similar regional variations have been reported from Vietnam, Sri Lanka, Turkey and Peru.[9–12]

Inequalities in child mortality

Figure 5.6 starkly and graphically illustrates inequalities related to income in New Delhi.[1]

Data from Bangladesh in 1975 showed that the death rate for children from one to four years of age varied from 85.5/1000 in landless families to 17.5/1000 in those families owning three or more acres.[13] Table 5.5 is based on Costa Rican data collected between 1968 and 1969. The familiar pattern of mortality differences is demonstrated between different social groups classified according to father's occupation.

Further evidence comes from a more recent study carried out in urban and rural areas of Bangladesh and Pakistan (*see* Table 5.6).[14] The results of this study indicate the relationship between socio-economic factors and child mortality, but also

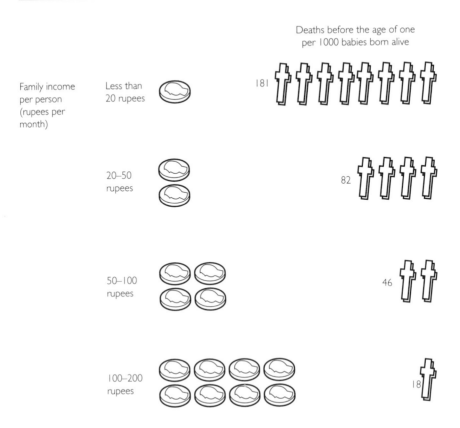

Figure 5.6 'A living wage' – the relationship between family income and infant death in a New Delhi study. (Source [1])

raise the important possibility that the effect of variables may differ according to the setting. It is likely that this reflects the ability of the variable to act as a reliable proxy for socio-economic status in different settings.

Many other studies have confirmed that mortality outcomes for children in less developed countries vary with socio-economic status.[10,12,15,17] Other studies have focused on the relationship between mortality and maternal education.[18,19] In a Bangladeshi study, Bhuiya and Streatfield report that the odds of dying were highest for children of mothers with no formal education (1.86) and higher for children of mothers having only primary-level education (1.43) compared with the children of mothers

Table 5.5   Child mortality rates in Costa Rica classified by the father's occupation, 1968–69. (Source [27])

Social class	Number of deaths between birth and age two per 1000 births
High and middle bourgeoisie	20
Middle class	39
Proletariat	80
Agricultural workers	99
Average	80

with secondary education.[20] The results of a Brazilian cohort study are shown in Table 5.7.[21]

Majumder and Islam demonstrate a clear link between maternal and paternal education levels and child mortality.[22]

Maternal education in many less developed countries is intimately linked with socio-economic circumstances and is a reasonable proxy for socio-economic position. Victora and co-workers demonstrate this link in data from Brazil, which are summarised in Table 5.8.[21]

In both Bangladesh and Pakistan, maternal and paternal education levels are closely correlated with housing and wealth.[14] The relationship of education and income is considered below as part of the causal debate as well as in Part Three.

Inequalities in child morbidity and growth

Malnutrition is the single most important factor in childhood mortality and morbidity in the less developed countries; it is estimated that more than 200 million of the world's children are inadequately nourished, of whom 10 million suffer severe malnutrition.[1] Malnutrition is unevenly distributed between countries (*see* Chapter 2, p. 29).

Malnutrition affects individuals and populations through a cyclical process, which is illustrated in Figure 5.7.

The mother whose growth is stunted as a result of childhood malnutrition is likely to produce a low birth weight infant, who then goes on to experience further undernutrition and poor growth, leading to stunting and perpetuation of the cycle.

Table 5.6 Adjusted* odds ratios (95% confidence intervals) for variables predictive of child death in urban and rural communities in Bangladesh and Pakistan. (Source [14] p. 1295)

Bangladesh		Pakistan	
Urban	*Rural*	*Urban*	*Rural*
Landless 1.39 (0.85–2.25)	Uneducated mother 2.32 (1.31–4.09)	Uneducated mother 1.28 (0.86–1.90)	Landless 6.13 (1.57–23.88)
Manual occupation 2.18 (1.29–3.68)	Earth floor 0.16 (0.04–0.61)	Manual occupation 1.44 (0.91–2.29)	Manual occupation 1.90 (0.29–12.62)
Earth floor 1.77 (1.10–2.84)	No. live births 1.79 (1.58–2.02)	No household water tap 1.38 (0.89–2.14)	No electricity 0.30 (0.10–0.89)
Rented house 1.80 (1.10–2.96)		Few possessions 2.00 (1.31–3.08)	Few possessions 2.39 (0.90–6.34)
No. live births 1.78 (1.59–2.01)		No. live births 1.66 (1.52–1.83)	No. live births 1.50 (1.25–1.80)

* Adjusted for all other variables retained in the model in each community; variables were retained in a forward stepwise procedure if significant at < 0.25; all variables retained in each community are included in this table.

Table 5.7   Association of maternal education with child health outcomes in Brazil. (Source [21])

Indices	Years of schooling				P
	0	1–4	5–8	9+	
Birthweight (g)					
<2000	6%	4%	3%	2%	<0.001
2000–	8%	6%	7%	5%	
2500–	26%	26%	24%	19%	
3000–	32%	36%	38%	39%	
3500+	28%	27%	28%	35%	
Mean	3082	3131	3160	3271	<0.001
	(335)	(1669)	(2502)	(1505)	
Perinatal mortality rate per 1000 births	36	39	35	19	0.007
	(335)	(1669)	(2502)	(1505)	
Infant mortality rate per 1000 live births	95	51	37	17	<0.001
	(283)	(1497)	(2299)	(1346)	
Hospital admissions from birth to age 20 months					
None	53%	62%	71%	87%	<0.001
Diarrhoea only	12%	11%	7%	3%	
Pneumonia only	13%	12%	8%	4%	
Diar. and pneum.	5%	3%	2%	0%	
Other causes	17%	12%	12%	6%	
	(249)	(1352)	(2126)	(1275)	
Mean length-for-age*	1.30	1.06	0.70	–0.15	<0.001
	(238)	(1352)	(2100)	(1270)	
Mean weight-for-age*	–0.77	–0.60	–0.29	0.22	<0.001
	(239)	(1325)	(2100)	(1270)	
Mean weight-for-length*	–0.02	0.02	0.17	0.43	<0.001
	(238)	(1324)	(2099)	(1268)	

* Expressed as mean z-scores of the US National Center for Health Statistics reference.

Table 5.8   Maternal education and potential confounding
variables in Brazil (Source [21])

	Years of schooling				Number of children	P
	0	1–4	5–8	9+		
Monthly family income (US$)	%	%	%	%		
≤50	13	48	36	3	1321 (100%)	<0.001
51–150	5	31	50	14	2866 (100%)	
151–300	2	12	44	42	1105 (100%)	
301–500	0	4	21	76	383 (100%)	
501+	0	1	8	91	336 (100%)	
Race						
White	5	25	42	28	4930 (100%)	<0.001
Non-white	9	38	40	12	1081 (100%)	
Maternal age (yr)						
<20	5	36	50	9	921 (100%)	<0.001
20–24	4	26	47	23	1868 (100%)	
25–29	4	25	38	34	1623 (100%)	
30–34	8	25	35	31	995 (100%)	
35–39	10	32	34	24	457 (100%)	
40+	22	33	29	16	147 (100%)	
Maternal height (m)						
<1.50	18	14	10	6	547 (100%)	<0.001
1.50–	35	30	28	17	1258 (100%)	
1.55	31	31	33	35	1970 (100%)	
1.60–	13	18	20	26	1594 (100%)	
1.65+	3	6	8	16	642 (100%)	
Schooling of husband/partner (yr)						
None	20	52	26	2	206 (100%)	<0.001
1–4	10	47	37	6	1111 (100%)	
5–8	3	26	54	17	2067 (100%)	
9+	0	7	31	63	1298 (100%)	

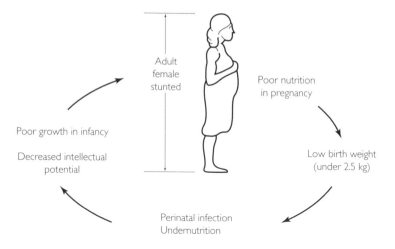

Figure 5.7   The cycle of malnutrition. (Source [1])

Malnutrition has a direct effect on growth: *wasting* occurs when the child's weight is less than expected for their height and is the result of short-term nutritional stress, and *stunting* entails the retardation in linear growth as measured by total body length or height, and results from long-term, chronic undernutrition.[23] Malnutrition also makes the child more susceptible to infection, and infection in its turn can exacerbate malnutrition.[1] Data from the Philippines suggest a strong correlation of non-verbal intelligence at age eight with stunting at age two, such that non-stunted children have scores 11 points higher than the most stunted. ([3] p. 16)

The evidence suggests that malnutrition is maldistributed within as well as between countries. A study in the Philippines reports a clear relationship between household income and nutritional status of children: children in households whose total income in the previous 12 months was 5700 pesos (US$626) or less are 38% more likely to suffer at least mild malnutrition than children in households reporting incomes of at least 23 400 pesos (US$2571), and are nearly 77% more likely to be moderately or severely malnourished.[24] Studies that have looked at wasting (reduced weight for height) and stunting (reduced linear growth) confirm the relationship with household income and socio-economic factors: in a birth cohort study in Pelotas,

Southern Brazil, Victora and co-workers report a significant effect of income on mean length-for-age, mean weight-for-age and mean weight-for-length, although the effect is modified by level of maternal education;[21] Forman and co-workers, reporting the results of the Bedouin Infant Feeding Study, found stunting in 19% of infants from low SES families compared with 12% in middle SES families and 5% in high SES families.[25] In a study of hospitalised children in Addis Ababa, Ethiopia, in 1985, children from low SES groups had weight-for-length scores of 87% of the median value of the standard compared with those from high SES groups, who had scores of 105% of the median value of the standard.[26]

Famine is the most acute and, in the age of television, the most visible form of malnutrition affecting populations. Children suffer most as a result of famine. Contrary to common belief, famines are not random 'acts of God', nor is food shortage a necessary prerequisite.[27,28] Famines can occur in the presence of abundant food supplies and it is the poor who have no 'food entitlement' who suffer the most devastating consequences.[28]

Using height attained at various ages, the relationship between growth and socio-economic factors is clearly demonstrated.[23] Figure 5.8 represents the differential in height attained at seven years of age between boys of high and low socio-economic status in various countries.

It is interesting to note from these data that children from high SES groups in most countries achieve mean heights equivalent to the 50th centile on the US National Center for Health Statistics (NCHS) growth charts derived from the US child population. As is discussed in detail in Chapter 7, these findings suggest that differences in growth observed between ethnic groups may be related as much to socio-economic as biological factors.

A study in East Africa demonstrates the same differences in mean heights attained between the ages of three and 13 years between privileged and underprivileged Bantu children, leading the authors to conclude that:

> *Poverty, poor food intakes, infectious and parasitic diseases and other environmental factors combine to prevent children from realising their growth potential.*[29]

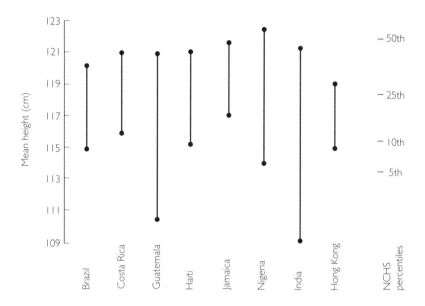

Figure 5.8 Mean heights of seven-year-old boys of high and low socio-economic status in various countries. (Source [23])

Twenty per cent of the underprivileged children in this study could not be plotted on the NCHS weight-for-height charts because their stature was below the lower end of the percentile distribution marked on the charts.

Amongst the poor in Lahore, Pakistan, differential rates of stunting have been reported: 63% of children aged 24 months in a peri-urban slum area showed stunting against reference values based on upper middle class Pakistani children compared with 54% in a village and 26% in an urban slum.[30] Poor children in the same study were delayed approximately three months in walking and fine motor skills compared with their upper middle class peers whose developmental progress was equivalent to that of reference European and North American populations.[31]

As would be expected from the cyclical process illustrated in Figure 5.7, low birth weight in less developed countries is closely correlated with socio-economic status.[1] Malnourished mothers in poor communities fail to gain weight adequately

Table 5.9   Relationship of mean birth weight to socio-economic status in various less developed countries. (Source [1])

Place	Population	Subject (socio-economic status)	Mean birth weight (g)
Madras	Indian	Well-to-do	2985
		Mostly poor	2736
South India	Indian	Wealthy	3182
		Poor	2810
Bombay	Indian	Upper class	3247
		Lower middle class	2796
		Lower class	2578
Ghana	African	Prosperous	3188
		General population	2879
Tanzania	African	Upper class	3150
		Lower class	2700
Indonesia	Javanese	Well-to-do	3022
		Poor	2816
Britain	National cohort	Social class I–II	3380
	1958	Social class V	3290

during pregnancy and the fetus is therefore susceptible to growth retardation.[32] Table 5.9 compares mean birth weights by SES groups in various countries.

As in developed countries (*see* Chapter 6), low birth weight is the most important factor in perinatal and infant mortality. Figure 5.9 is derived from the results of a large Indian study and shows the importance of birth weight as a determinant of infant mortality.[1]

Much of the childhood morbidity and mortality in less developed countries is linked with poverty through low birth weight and the cycle of malnutrition (Figure 5.7). For a classification of the most important diseases affecting children in less developed countries, *see* Table 4.6 in Chapter 4.

Specific nutritional diseases such as iron-deficiency anaemia, vitamin A deficiency and rickets (vitamin D deficiency) have an obvious and direct relationship to undernutrition. Vitamin A deficiency is associated with increased susceptibility to infection: in three separate trials of children hospitalised with measles,

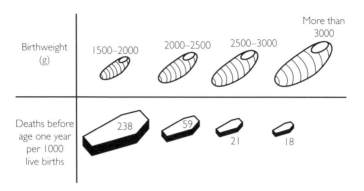

Figure 5.9 Relationship between birth weight and infant mortality in India. (Source [1])

deaths among children given high-dose vitamin A supplements were significantly lower than among children not supplemented. ([3] p. 72) Iron-deficiency anaemia is reported to be present in 59% of pregnant women in less developed countries compared with 14% in developed countries.[33] Iron deficiency and zinc deficiency also appear to be important for the body's first-line defences by maintaining the physical barriers of skin and mucosa that prevent organisms from invading the body and enhancing leucocyte and macrophage activity. ([3] p. 73)

Airborne communicable diseases such as measles and whooping cough occur more frequently in poor children. Whooping cough is spread by droplet infection and the chances of infection in early infancy, associated with increased severity, are enhanced by overcrowding and inadequate housing.

The most infamous disease of poverty, TB, is making a resurgence across the world affecting developed (*see* Chapter 6) and less developed countries, and is now the fourth biggest cause of death, killing 20 000 people a year.[34] Up to 39% of Filipino children between five and nine years of age living in the country's slums are infected which is twice the national average.[34] As in the developed world in the 19th century (Chapter 4), cramped, overcrowded and poorly ventilated housing and malnutrition contribute to the spread of the disease. The social conditions predisposing to the spread of the disease and the problems related to treatment access have been described by one author as 'political violence' – the systematic destruction of human life as a result of structural inequalities.[35]

Acute rheumatic fever (ARF) is another disease associated with poverty and overcrowding which was prevalent in many developed countries until relatively recently. A recent study from a hospital in Bangladesh suggests that ARF continues to have a strong association with socio-economic disadvantage: children from households with low income, poor living conditions and substandard housing were all at increased risk of admission for ARF.[36]

Of the water-related and faecally transmitted diseases, diarrhoea is the most important cause of childhood morbidity and mortality. Across the world, children under five years of age are estimated to suffer one billion episodes of diarrhoea annually; the individual child in an urban slum community experiences an average of four episodes of diarrhoea per year, with a range from two to 12.[1,37] Diarrhoea particularly affects weanlings and infants who are bottle-fed and is closely linked to the absence of clean water and sanitation.[4] Poor children suffer more episodes of diarrhoea in less developed countries, though within poor communities marked variations in diarrhoea episodes are not explained by socio-economic differences.[38] Possible reasons for these contradictory findings are considered below.

Washing and bathing in dirty water are responsible for the incidence of many communicable diseases: at least 100 million children aged five to 14 years of age are infected with schistosomiasis, and children living in poor environments are the most vulnerable.

Human immunodeficiency virus (HIV) infection leading to acquired immune deficiency syndrome (AIDS) has become one of the most important causes of morbidity and mortality in parts of Africa and other countries, developed and less developed. Evidence is emerging that its worst effects are seen in poor communities, particularly those affected by migrant labour systems leading to prolonged separation of men from their wives and families.[39] Thus poor children are likely to suffer the worst consequences in terms of loss of life and loss of parents.

Explanations of child health inequalities in less developed countries

The causal debate related to health inequalities is considered in detail in Part Three. This short section is part of that debate but I feel that this chapter would be incomplete and one-sided without some consideration of these important questions as they relate to less developed countries. In common with Chapters 4 and 6, the main purpose of this chapter is to examine the evidence for health inequalities in some detail as well as to establish the universal nature of the phenomenon. Thus far, explanations have not been considered.

As with the debate in developed countries, the dominant and opposing schools of thought are the structural and the behavioural (*see* Part Three): the structural school maintains that health inequalities arise as a result of differences in the socio-economic structure of society which lead to poverty and its health consequences; the behavioural school holds that cultural and behavioural patterns associated with and contributing to poverty explain much of the observed difference in health outcomes. The artefact and social mobility explanations (*see* Part Three) which have been advanced in developed countries do not seem to have gained any currency in relation to less developed countries. Maternal education is universally accepted as an important determinant of child health in less developed countries. It has been variously claimed by both schools: in many studies it is taken as the main indicator of SES, whilst in others it is seen as a marker of cultural level and as an explanation of observed SES differences in child health outcomes.

Though the evidence on an international, national, regional and individual level is strong for the key role of SES factors in child health outcomes, there have been a number of studies which have failed to demonstrate SES differences in child health outcomes in less developed countries.[7,8,38,40] In a study of two major population centres in Southern Sudan, income was eliminated as a key factor by logistic regression analysis and the positive associations for child mortality were found to be immunisation, maternal education and oral rehydration therapy.[7]

In Southern Peru, other cultural practices such as infanticide –
particularly affecting female offspring – as well as parental
education are suggested as possible determinants of child mortality, whereas land ownership was found to have little or no
effect.[40] Bailey and co-workers, in their study of infant mortality in rural North-east Brazil, state: 'post-neonatal survival
depends largely on factors relating to child care, whilst neonatal deaths are more likely to be associated with biological
factors'.[8] A further study in Bangladesh shows a relationship
between childhood mortality and income but the relationship
is curvilinear, with children of middle income families enjoying
the lowest mortality rates.[20]

All the above-mentioned studies have emphasised the
importance of cultural and educational factors in determining
child health, and have tended to suggest that socio-economic
factors may be less important or explained by behavioural
factors. McCance is forthright in his explanation of malnutrition when he states:

> *The fundamental trouble in the underdeveloped parts
> of the world is the illiteracy and the absence of all the
> 'know how' and services that the western nations have
> built for themselves. Even after arriving in this country
> (the UK), West Indian women may be 'incredibly
> helpless, disinterested and ignorant of the baby's most
> elementary needs'. Serious setbacks usually do not
> begin before the mother weans the baby and the earlier
> this is done the earlier the child is likely to get into
> difficulties. Dirty vessels, infected cow's milk, if the
> child is given any, or other foods if it is not, lead to
> gastroenteritis, sometimes quite mild, which the mother
> treats by the light of nature and often produces the
> starvation or protein deficiency herself.* ([41] pp. 500–1)

Aside from the obvious racist overtones, this statement clearly
places the responsibility for infant diarrhoea and malnutrition
on the mother. His chapter details many studies which highlight
the role of cultural factors in the causation of malnutrition.
Only in relation to child health in Johannesburg and South

India (p. 502) does he acknowledge the role of poverty, and even then his emphasis is on maternal ignorance as the primary determinant.

Others have argued that this interpretation of maternal responsibility through her own ignorance and that of her culture ignores the social setting of maternal illiteracy. Palloni places illiteracy within a social context and states:

> The extent of illiteracy in a society reflects not only the limitations of individuals but, more importantly, the capacity of a system to organise and mobilise to fulfil societal necessities. From this point of view the proportion illiterate in a population is less an indication of the fraction of mothers with inadequate knowledge to treat and feed a sick infant or to challenge the authority of elders than a reflection of the degree of social and political maturity of the system above and beyond the amounts of wealth at its disposal and the degree of equality of its distribution. ([42] pp. 642–3)

To illustrate this point he uses data gathered in Latin America (*see* Table 5.10). This shows that although improvements in mortality are related to the mother's education, the amount of improvement varies widely by country. The author concludes that the effects of maternal education on child mortality are contingent on social setting, and a disadvantageous setting is more severely felt at the lowest levels of education, although it operates at all levels.

Hertz and co-workers conclude from the results of a cross-national comparison of social and environmental factors and mortality rates:

> The overall successes (of particular countries) indicate that better health and nutrition is produced by the synergistic action of improved sanitation, higher education levels, controlled overpopulation and more equitable distribution of economic resources, better housing, increased investment, higher wages and generally more extensive welfare services. ([43] p. 113)

Table 5.10   Probability of dying during the first two years of life by education of mother in different Latin American countries (calculated from 1970s data). (Source [42] p. 643)

Country	Years of education of mother						Average slope
	Total	0	1–3	4–6	7–9	10+	
Cuba	41	46	45	34	29		5.67
Paraguay	75	104	80	61	45	27	19.25
Costa Rica	81	125	98	70	51	33	23.00
Colombia	88	126	95	63	42	32	23.50
Chile	91	131	108	92	66	46	21.25
Dominican Republic	123	172	130	106	81	54	29.50
Ecuador	127	176	134	101	61	46	35.00
Honduras	140	171	129	99	60	35	34.00
El Salvador	145	158	142	111	58	30	32.00
Guatemala	149	169	135	85	58	44	31.25
Nicaragua	149	168	142	115	73	48	30.00
Peru	169	207	136	102	77	70	34.30
Bolivia	202	245	209	176	110		45.00
Argentina	58	96	75	59	39	26	16.80

Other authors reach similar conclusions from cross-national studies.[44,45] Studies in single countries have shown the close association between education and wealth and have suggested that low socio-economic levels are directly related to the mother's poor capability of intervention during her infant's illness as well as poor knowledge about vaccinations and non-use of growth charts.[10,14,46] It has been suggested that failure to relate socio-economic factors to child health outcomes in rural studies such as those listed above may result from the fact that poverty is so widespread in rural areas that it is undifferentiated in its effect on child health outcomes, and/or the economic variables themselves are inadequately defined and insensitive to economic variation among rural families.[17]

In summary, there is strong evidence of child health inequalities in less developed countries. Many variables, other than SES, have been implicated, the main one of which is maternal education. However, maternal education is itself closely related to SES and will act as a powerful confounding variable in any analysis of the relationship between SES and child health outcomes (*see* Part Three). It seems most appropriate to consider the synergism between these factors rather than try to identify which is the more powerful and which explains the other. The construction of causal pathways is the most interesting approach to this problem.[45,48,49] This approach is considered in more detail in Part Three.

Summary

1   There is a strong association between GNP per capita and child health outcomes.

2   Less developed countries with low GNP per capita can achieve good child health outcomes by strategies which minimise income disparities, increase maternal literacy and improve nutritional levels of the population.

3   Marked regional differences in child health outcomes are evident in many less developed countries which relate to the relative socio-economic status of the region.

4   Marked differences are found in childhood mortality and morbidity between different socio-economic groups within less developed countries.

5   A synergistic relationship between maternal education, socio-economic circumstances and various cultural factors would seem to best explain observed differences in child health outcomes in less developed countries.

References

1   Ebrahim GJ (1985) *Social and Community Paediatrics in Developing Countries*. Macmillan, London.

2   United Nations Development Programme (1994) *Human Development Report 1994*. UNDP & Oxford University Press, New York.

3 Bellamy C (1998) *The State of the World's Children*. Oxford University Press, New York.

4 Grant J (1994) *The State of the World's Children*. Oxford University Press, New York.

5 Knight J and Song L (1999) *Increasing Wage Inequality in China: Efficiency versus Equity?* Applied Economics Discussion Paper, No. 211, Institute of Economics and Statistics, University of Oxford.

6 Tung-liang Chang (1999) Economic transition and changing relations between income inequality and mortality in Taiwan: regression analysis. *BMJ*. **319**:1162–5.

7 Roth EA and Balan Karup K (1990) Child mortality levels and survival patterns from southern Sudan. *J. Biosoc. Sci.* **22**:365–72.

8 Bailey P, Ong Tsui A, Janowitz B *et al.* (1990) A study of infant mortality and causes of death in a rural north-east Brazilian community. *J. Biosoc. Sci.* **22**:349–63.

9 Svenson IE, Thang NM, San PB *et al.* (1993) Factors influencing infant mortality in Vietnam. *J. Biosoc. Sci.* **25**:285–302.

10 Waxler NE, Morrison BM, Sirisena WM *et al.* (1985) Infant mortality in Sri Lankan households: a causal model. *Soc. Sci. Med.* **20**:381–92.

11 Dedeoglu N (1990) Health and social inequities in Turkey. *Soc. Sci. Med.* **31**:387–92.

12 Edmonston B and Andes N (1983) Community variations in infant and child mortality in Peru. *J. Epidemiol. Community Health*. **37**:121–6.

13 Sanders D (1985) *The Struggle for Health*. Macmillan Education, London.

14 Durkin MS, Islam S, Hasan ZM *et al.* (1994) Measures of socioeconomic status for child health research: comparative

results from Bangladesh and Pakistan. *Soc. Sci. Med.* **38**:1289–97.

15 Woods CH (1982) The political economy of infant mortality in Sao Paulo, Brazil. *Int. J. Health Services.* **12**:215–29.

16 Shah NM and Shah MA (1990) Socioeconomic and health-care determinants of child survival in Kuwait. *J. Biosoc. Sci.* **22**:239–53.

17 Millard AV (1985) Child mortality and economic variation among rural Mexican households. *Soc. Sci. Med.* **20**:589–99.

18 Caldwell J (1979) Education as a factor in mortality decline: an examination of Nigerian data. *Popul. Stud.* **33**:395–413.

19 Hobcraft JN, McDonald JW and Rutstein SO (1984) Socioeconomic factors in infant and child mortality: a cross-national comparison. *Popul. Stud.* **38**:193–223.

20 Bhuiya A and Streatfield K (1992) A hazard logit model analysis of covariates of childhood mortality in Matlab, Bangladesh. *J. Biosoc. Sci.* **24**:447–62.

21 Victora CG, Huttly SRA, Barros FC *et al.* (1992) Maternal education in relation to early and late child health outcomes: findings from a Brazilian cohort study. *Soc. Sci. Med.* **34**:899–905.

22 Majumder AK and Islam SMS (1993) Socioeconomic and environmental determinants of child survival in Bangladesh. *J. Biosoc. Sci.* **25**:311–18.

23 Martorell R (1984) Genetics, environment and growth: issues in the assessment of nutritional status. In *Genetic Factors in Nutrition* (eds A Velasquez and H Bourges). Academic Press, New York.

24 Magnani RJ, Mock NB, Bertrand WE *et al.* (1993) Breast-feeding, water and sanitation and childhood malnutrition in the Philippines. *J. Biosoc. Sci.* **25**:195–211.

25   Forman MR, Guptill KS, Chang DN *et al.* (1990) Under-nutrition among Bedouin Arab infants: the Bedouin Infant Feeding Study. *Am. J. Clin. Nutr.* **51**:343–9.

26   Groenewald WGF and Tilahun M (1990) Anthropometric indicators of nutritional status, socioeconomic factors and mortality in hospitalized children in Addis Ababa. *J. Biosoc. Sci.* **22**:373–9.

27   Gray A (ed.) (1993) *World Health and Disease.* Open University Press, Milton Keynes.

28   Scrimshaw NS (1987) The phenomenon of famine. *Annu. Rev. Nutr.* **7**:1–21.

29   Stephensen LS, Lathan MC and Jansen A (1983) *A comparison of growth standards: similarities between NCHS, Harvard, Denver and privileged African children and differences with Kenyan rural children.* Cornell International Nutrition Monograph Series, No. 12, Cornell University, New York.

30   Karlberg J, Ashraf RN, Saleemi M *et al.* (1993) Early child health in Lahore, Pakistan. 11: Growth. *Acta Paediatr.* **82**(10):S119–49.

31   Yaqoob M, Ferngren H, Jalil F *et al.* (1993). Early child health in Lahore, Pakistan. 12: Milestones. *Acta Paediatr.* **82**(10):S151–7.

32   Ebrahim GJ (1982) *Child Health in a Changing Environment.* Macmillan, London.

33   DeMaeyer E and Adiels-Tegman M (1985) The prevalence of anaemia in the world. *Who Stat. Q.* **38**:302–16.

34   Wallerstein C (1999) Tuberculosis ravages Philippine slums. *BMJ.* **319**:402.

35   Farmer P (1997) Social scientists and the new tuberculosis. *Soc. Sci. Med.* **44**:347–58.

36 Zaman MM, Yoshiike N, Chowdhury AH *et al.* (1997) Socio-economic deprivation associated with acute rheumatic fever. A hospital-based case–control study in Bangladesh. *Paediatr. Perinat. Epidemiol.* **11**:322–32.

37 Snyder JD and Merson MH (1982) The magnitude of the global problem of acute diarrhoeal disease: a review of active surveillance data. *Bull. WHO.* **60**:605–13.

38 Moy RJD, Booth IW, Choto RGA *et al.* (1991) Risk factors for high diarrhoea frequency: a study of rural Zimbabwe. *Trans Roy. Soc. Trop. Med. Hyg.* **85**:814–18.

39 Sanders D and Sambo A (1991) AIDS in Africa: the implications of economic recession and structural adjustment. *Health Policy Plann.* **6**:157–65.

40 de Meer K, Bergman R and Kusner JS (1993) Socio-cultural determinants of child mortality in southern Peru: including some methodological considerations. *Soc. Sci. Med.* **36**:317–31.

41 McCance RA (1971) Malnutrition in the children of underdeveloped countries. In *Recent Advances in Paediatrics, No. 4* (eds D Hull and D Gairdner). Churchill Livingstone, Edinburgh.

42 Palloni A (1981) Mortality in Latin America: emerging patterns. *Popul. Dev. Rev.* **7**:623–48.

43 Hertz E, Hebert JR and Landon J (1994) Social and environmental factors and life expectancy, infant mortality and maternal mortality rates: results of a cross-national comparison. *Soc. Sci. Med.* **39**:105–14.

44 Stanton B (1994) Child health: equity in the non-industrialized countries. *Soc. Sci. Med.* **38**:1375–81.

45 Millard AV (1994) Child mortality and economic variation among rural Mexican households. *Soc. Sci. Med.* **20**:589–99.

46 Mosley WH (1985) Will primary care reduce infant and child mortality? A critique of some current strategies with

special references to Africa and Asia. In *Selected Readings in the Cultural, Social and Behavioural Determinants of Health* (eds J Caldwell and G Santow). Highland Press, Canberra, Australia.

47   Cortinovas I, Vella V and Ndiku J (1993) Construction of a socioeconomic index to facilitate analysis of health data in developing countries. *Soc. Sci. Med.* **36**:1087–97.

48   Waxler NE, Morrison BM, Sirisena WM *et al.* (1985) Infant mortality in Sri Lankan households: a causal model. *Soc. Sci. Med.* **20**:381–92.

49   Frisch AS, Kallen DJ, Griffore RJ *et al.* (1992) Social variances and infant survival: a path analysis approach. *J. Biosoc. Sci.* **24**:175–83.

6

Poverty and child health in developed countries

Introduction

The two preceding chapters have demonstrated the relationship between 'absolute' poverty and child health. Chapter 4 shows that, prior to the rapid improvement in living standards in what are now called the developed countries, the health experience of children was similar to that in less developed countries today. Chapters 4 and 5 confirm the existence of marked inequalities in child health closely linked to socioeconomic circumstances in societies in which absolute poverty affects a significant proportion of the population, and the greater the proportion of the population living in absolute poverty the worse the child health outcomes. By contrast, children from high income families living in such societies experience health outcomes compatible with those of children living in developed countries.

This chapter considers the effects of 'relative' poverty in developed countries on child health. The relationship between relative poverty and child health has often been considered ahistorically and with a narrow focus on the experience in a particular country. By linking the evidence with that presented in the two preceding chapters and drawing on data from as broad a range of developed countries as possible, I have attempted to demonstrate the continuity of child poverty and its health effects over time and across national boundaries.

Mortality rates are the traditional measure of the health status of a population group and the infant mortality rate

(IMR) – deaths in the first year of life per thousand live births – has been used as a proxy for a country's general health status (*see* Chapters 3 and 4).[1] The effects of socio-economic status (SES) on death in childhood are considered using data from different developed countries. Available data linking childhood morbidity, birth weight and growth and SES are considered, followed by an assessment of the effects of SES on educational attainment, life quality and self-esteem. Evidence for increasing disparity in child health between socio-economic groups in developed countries is examined and, in a concluding section, the significance of the evidence in the context of the health effects of relative poverty will be discussed.

Mortality

Deaths in infancy

All developed countries have experienced a remarkable reduction in IMR in the last 100 years (Figure 6.1). The rate of fall has varied from country to country but the trend has been consistently downwards. Medical advances have made some contribution but the trend long preceded the most important advances of the 20th century (for example, neonatal intensive care) and owes more to improvements in living standards than medical advances.[2,3]

The fall in IMR has affected all social groups though, as Figure 6.2 shows. In England and Wales the difference between the most and least privileged as represented by the Registrar General's Social Class (RGSC), a measure of the occupation of the head of the household (*see* Chapter 1), has remained remarkably constant.

Most deaths in childhood in developed countries occur in the first year of life, with the neonatal period being the most vulnerable. Infant mortality rates show consistent differences by SES across countries. The data for England and Wales in Table 6.1 show an increased risk of infant death for children of unskilled worker families compared with children of professional families.[4] The risk is even higher for those infants of

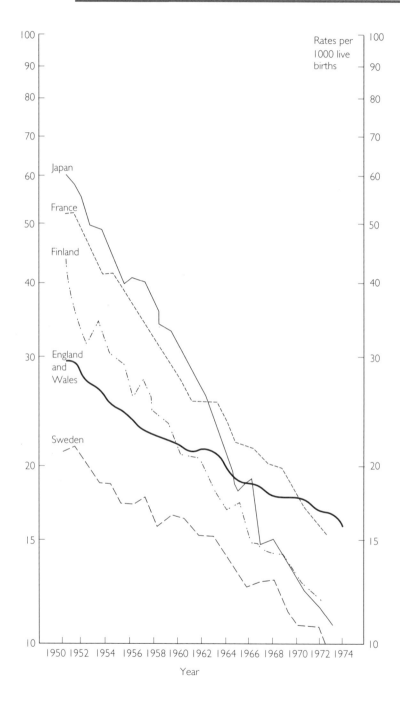

Figure 6.1   Fall in IMR in developed countries.

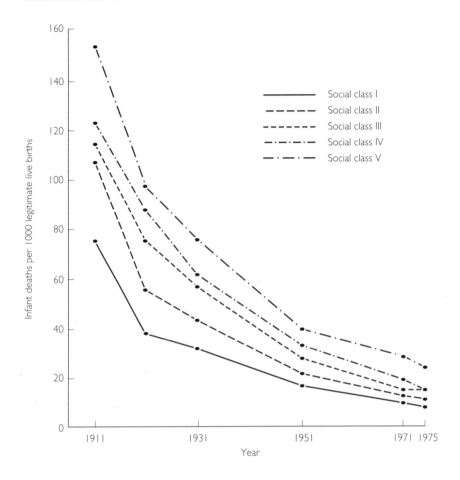

Figure 6.2 Social class trends in IMR at four Census dates, 1911–71, England and Wales. (Source [78] p. 239)

families classified as 'Other'. The trend is the same as that shown in Figure 6.2, with continuing reduction in IMR across all social groups but persistence of social difference.

UK regional differences in IMRs, varying between 6.8/1000 live births in the South West and 9.9/1000 live births in the West Midlands in 1990, reflect socio-economic differences as well as differences in IMR by ethnic minority group (*see* also Chapter 7).[5] Ethnic group and regional differences are marked in the USA: in the late 1980s, black American infants were

Table 6.1   Infant deaths by father's social class – England and Wales, 1987–90 (within, and jointly registered outside, marriage). (Source [4] p. 103)

Social class	1987–88 rate	1987–89 rate	1988–90 rate
All	8.5	8.3	7.9
I	7.0	6.7	6.2
II	6.7	6.6	6.2
IIIN	7.3	7.3	7.1
IIIM	8.3	8.0	7.6
IV	9.9	10.0	9.5
V	12.1	11.8	11.7
Ratio V/I	1.73	1.76	1.89
Other	13.8	13.7	14.3

twice as likely to die in the first year of life (*see* also Chapter 7), and in the 1975–77 period IMRs varied from 12.8 in New England and the Pacific to 16.9 in the South Atlantic.[6,7] For white Americans in the mid-1980s, the rates varied from 7.9 in New Jersey to 11.3 in Idaho.[6] Danziger and Stern, and Wise and Meyers argue that these ethnic and regional differences reflect the SES of the ethnic groups and the regions and they report a correlation between a state's poverty rate and the IMR of its white American infants.[6,8]

Table 6.2 shows trends in regional differences in IMR in Italy. As with the UK and US regional data, these differences reflect socio-economic variation between the regions: in 1985, the average income of families in the north and central regions was 24.7% higher than in the south and the islands, and chances of a child living in poverty in the south and the islands, were greater than for the other regions.[9] Similar regional differences have been reported from the former USSR in 1988, where the IMR varied from 11 in Lithuania to 53 in Turkmenistan.[10]

Data from the Italian Central Institute of Statistics in 1975 confirm the expected gradient in IMR by maternal education: 23.7/1000 live births for mothers with no education or primary school only compared with 9.2 /1000 for mothers with college education.[11]

Table 6.2   Perinatal and infant mortality rates by Italian region, 1980 and 1985. (Source [9])

	Stillbirths			*Perinatal mortality*			*Infant mortality*		
	1980	*1985*	*1987*	*1980*	*1985*	*1987*	*1980*	*1985*	*1987*
North-West	7.4	5.9		16.1	12.6		12.4	8.4	
North-East	6.7	5.4		14.6	11.6		12.0	7.9	
Centre	7.5	5.6		15.6	12.9		12.2	9.0	
South/Islands	9.3	7.8		19.9	15.7		16.5	12.4	
Italy	8.2	6.6	6.2	17.5	13.2	12.4	14.2	10.3	9.6

French data from 1970 show a risk of death for an infant of an unskilled worker of 2.49 compared with an infant of a professional.[12] Similar differential risks were reported for infants in Poland and Denmark during the same time period and a comprehensive literature review, involving 26 studies from the USA and Europe, concluded that strong differentials in IMR by SES persisted into the mid-1970s.[10,13] Data from urban Canada shows positive IMR gradients from the richest to the poorest neighbourhood income quintile from 10/1000 to 20/1000 in 1971 and 5/1000 to 8/1000 in 1991.[14]

Swedish data are of particular interest as Sweden has one of the lowest IMRs in the world and a long and relatively uninterrupted social policy of income redistribution (*see* also Chapter 10). Combining medical birth registration data for 1976–81 with census data for 1975–80, IMRs by socio-economic groups were calculated, showing an IMR of 5.9 in the highest socio-economic group compared to 7.2 in the lowest.[1] Elmen reports higher differentials between IMRs for high, medium and low income areas of the city of Goteborg in the period between 1981 and 1985: relative risk of infant death of 1.8 in medium and 2.0 in low income areas compared to high income areas.[15] Kohler concludes that 'infant and perinatal mortality in Sweden is still linked to socio-economic conditions, but less obviously than in most other countries'.[1]

Of equal interest are the former socialist countries of Eastern Europe. These were countries based on the concept of equality and equitable income distribution. However, as Table 6.3 shows, there were very marked differences in IMR between republics in former Yugoslavia in 1981, and these were closely related to each republic's per capita GNP. There was a fivefold disparity in IMR between the best (Slovenia) and the worst (Kosovo), which increased to a ninefold difference when post-neonatal mortality alone was considered.[16] In addition, there are marked differences within each republic reflecting socio-economic differences between areas: in Slovenia, IMR varies from 4/1000 in Kamnik to 33.7/1000 in Cernika, and in Kosovo from 30.5/1000 in Leposavic to 117.8/1000 in Kacanik.

Mastilica reports marked social class inequalities in former Yugoslavia and argues that these are in line with sociological studies which, despite the avowed commitment of the government to social equality, show a hierarchy of social groups with a political and managerial elite at the top and workers and peasants at the bottom.[16] A similar picture of marked regional and socio-economic variation in IMRs is reported from other former socialist countries of Eastern Europe: in Bulgaria, the IMR in urban areas was 13.9 in 1987 compared with 16.6 in rural areas; in Hungary, in 1987, IMR varied between 36.1 for the least educated mothers and 10.3 for the most educated; in Poland in 1987 the IMR for infants of the least educated mothers was almost twice that of the most educated.[17-19] In commenting on these findings from former socialist countries,

Table 6.3   IMRs and GNP per capita index by republics and provinces in former Yugoslavia, 1981. (Source [16] p. 406)

	IMR	GNP index
Slovenia	13.3	196
Croatia	18.9	126
Serbia proper	23.8	98
Vojvodina	17.1	118
Bosnia and Hercegovina	30.1	67
Montenegro	22.8	79
Macedonia	51.1	66
Kosovo	62.9	29
Yugoslavia	30.8	100

Wnuk-Lipinski and Illsley state: 'the empirical findings discussed in country profiles show that these unequal burdens (health inequalities) have clear class connotations although some other dimensions of social differentiation (gender, place of residence, region) may also be substantial'.[20]

Data relating perinatal mortality rates (PMR – stillbirths and deaths in the first month of life/1000 births) and the components of the IMR, neonatal mortality rate (NMR – deaths in the first month of life/1000 live births) and post-neonatal mortality rate (PNMR – deaths between one month and one year of age/1000 live births), to socio-economic circumstances are available from fewer countries. They demonstrate a similar social gradient.[1,21] Greek data show marked regional differences in PMR which are in part related to the economic standing of the region.[22] Perinatal mortality demonstrates a positive social gradient from least to most deprived for specific causes of death, including congenital anomalies.[23] The gradients disappear in infants less than 2500 g but persist in infants of higher birth weight. This finding is consistent with Leon's findings.[24] Similar gradients in cause-specific infant death rates were seen in England and Wales between 1990 and 1995 (Figure 6.3).[25]

The social gradient in sudden infant death syndrome is consistent over time and between countries: in a systematic

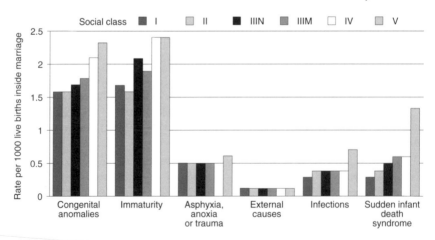

Figure 6.3   Infant mortality by social class of father (inside marriage only): selected causes of death, England and Wales, 1990–95. (Source [25] p. 88)

review of observational data of the relationship of socio-economic status to sudden unexpected death in infancy, 39 out of 40 studies over a 30-year period demonstrated a social gradient.[26] Recent studies, following the fall in sudden unexpected death in infancy (SUDI) rates in most industrial countries, indicate a sharper social gradient with deaths increasingly concentrated in the most disadvantaged groups.[27,28]

Deaths in childhood

In contrast to earlier historical periods (*see* Chapter 4) and less developed countries (*see* Chapter 5), deaths beyond the first year of life are now very unusual in developed countries. They are often associated with unnatural causes and accidents are now the commonest cause of death beyond one year of age.[29] However, the same socio-economic gradients noted for death in infancy are found in this age group, though evidence is available from fewer countries. For this reason the evidence presented here comes mainly from the UK and the USA.

All-cause mortality rates for England and Wales by age group (1–15 years; 1–4 years; 5–9 years; 10–14 years) and by gender for two periods, 1979–83 and 1991–93, are shown in Table 6.4.[25] Across the whole of childhood, despite the fall in mortality rates, the social differential in childhood deaths persists with twice as many children in social class V dying compared with social class I. The gradients are steepest at 1–4 years and for boys, especially in the 10–14 age group.

Though few children die after infancy, children from RGSC V families are twice as likely to die as those in RGSC I. Starfield and Budetti estimate that poor children in the USA are one and a half to three times more likely to die after the first year of life as non-poor children, and these disparities hold good for poor white American as well as poor black American children.[30] A study based on the Swedish Census-linked Deaths registry for the period 1980–86[31] reported a twofold increase in risk for all-cause mortality (0–12 years) among the children of poorest occupational groups compared with the children of non-manual families. The increased risk persisted after adjustment for gender,

Table 6.4   Childhood mortality rates (per 100 000) by age and gender, England and Wales. (Source [25] p. 92)

	Children		Boys		Girls	
	1979–80, 82–83	*1991–93*	*1979–80, 82–83*	*1991–93*	*1979–80, 82–83*	*1991–93*
Age 1–4						
I	34	27	34	34	34	21
II	34	23	35	24	32	22
IIIN	41	23	44	24	37	22
IIIM	47	37	53	40	42	33
IV	57	30	63	33	51	28
V	98	71	111	75	84	67
England & Wales	48	34	53	37	44	30
Age 5–9						
I	21	14	25	16	18	12
II	19	12	21	13	16	11
IIIN	22	11	25	13	19	7
IIIM	23	19	26	21	19	16
IV	28	14	32	16	23	13
V	42	30	51	34	31	26
England & Wales	25	16	29	18	20	14
Age 10–14						
I	19	14	21	15	16	13
II	19	13	23	14	16	12
IIIN	18	15	21	17	14	12
IIIM	23	22	26	25	19	18
IV	24	20	30	26	17	15
V	30	29	36	41	24	17
England & Wales	23	18	28	22	19	15
Age 1–15						
I	24	18	26	21	21	15
II	22	16	25	17	19	15
IIIN	25	16	28	19	21	14
IIIM	28	26	32	29	24	22
IV	33	22	38	26	27	19
V	49	42	57	49	40	35
England & Wales	30	23	35	26	25	19

family structure, immigrant status and population density of the place of residence.

Using the England and Wales data for 1979–83, Woodroffe and co-workers conclude that 'class gradients are not present for all causes of death, but there is no main cause for which children in lower classes have relatively low rates'.[21] However, the class gradients become very steep for specific causes of death in childhood. Mortality from all injuries shows a more than threefold difference (Figure 6.4), which becomes almost sevenfold when deaths due to traffic collision with a pedestrian (RGSC V 7.0/100 000 population compared with RGSC I 1.5/100 000 population) are analysed separately, and eightfold for deaths due to fire (RGSC V 2.6/100 000 compared with RGSC I 0.3/100 000). More recent data for 1991–93 show that deaths from injury and poisoning fell in each social class, but the differential between the social classes had widened because of a slower rate of decline in social classes IV and V compared with social classes I and II.[25] During the same period the death rate due to fire and flame decreased in social classes I and II but increased in social class IV and V.[25] The results of a study in the Northern Regional Health Authority of the UK of fatal childhood accidents involving head injuries show a 15-fold difference in mortality between the most deprived decile of local authority electoral wards and the least deprived decile.[32] Social class gradients are also clear in other than traumatic deaths: mortality in this age group from congenital anomalies is almost three times as high in RGSC V children as in RGSC I children (*see* Figure 6.4).

Wise and Meyers report that deaths from fire in the USA show the greatest disparity between poor and non-poor children, and a major influence of poverty on motor vehicle occupant mortality in children, as well as a similar social gradient in deaths due to traffic collision with a pedestrian, to that seen in the England and Wales data.[8] An important cause of mortality, even in young children, in the USA, hardly seen in the UK, is homicide, usually with firearms. The concentration of homicide deaths in poor communities is well documented.[1]

Re-analysis of the data for England and Wales presented above suggests that the exclusion of households unclassified in

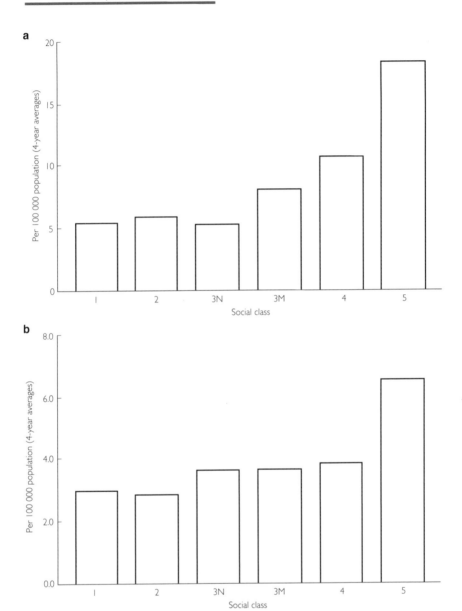

Figure 6.4   (a) Mortality from injuries age 1–14 years by social class, England and Wales, 1979–80 and 1982–83; (b) mortality from congenital anomalies age 1–14 years by social class, England and Wales, 1979–80 and 1982–83. (Source [21] p. 89, 90)

the RGSC significantly underestimates the social disparities in childhood deaths.[33] The authors identified a group of children whose parents were classified as 'unoccupied', largely consisting of economically inactive single mothers. This group constituted 6% (61 445 children) of all children – more than in either RGSC I or V. The age-specific mortality for this group was 68.8/100 000/year (1979–83) compared with 22.8 for RGSC I and 48.4 for RGSC V. Accidents and external causes of injury account for almost 60% of deaths in this group of children whose parents are classified as unoccupied.

Morbidity

Mortality has been and remains the mainstay of health status measurement within and between countries; however, as considered in Chapter 3, its limitations in countries where child deaths are rare have led to the search for more appropriate measures of health. Measures of morbidity can be divided broadly into two groups: medically defined morbidity and self-reported (or parent-reported) morbidity. Evidence linking medically defined and parent-reported morbidity and SES in developed countries is considered here.

Medically defined morbidity

There is a paucity of data relating specific diseases or medically defined conditions to SES. Where it exists, the social gradient tends to be the same as that noted for mortality with children in less favoured socio-economic circumstances experiencing greater levels of morbidity.

Bacterial meningitis, one of the life-threatening infections which remains relatively common among children in developed countries, has been shown to cluster in areas of deprivation and to be linked with poverty, overcrowding and low income.[30,34] *[smoking]* Acute rheumatic fever is rarely seen in most developed countries now but was a major cause of death and disability, particularly through its association with rheumatic heart disease.[35] Rheumatic fever and heart disease, when they occur, are closely related to socio-economic status and to membership of disadvantaged ethnic groups, such as the Aboriginals in Australia and Maoris and Pacific Islanders in New Zealand.[35-37]

Respiratory infections are the most frequent cause of ill health in children in developed countries, and pneumonia, like meningitis, remains a relatively common life-threatening illness. Data from the three UK National Cohort Studies,[38] in which cohorts of all children born during the same week across the country in 1946 (National Survey of Health and Development), 1958 (National Child Development Study) and 1970 (Child Health and Education Study) were followed, show a clear social class gradient in respiratory infection. A greater risk of upper and lower respiratory infection was found in lower

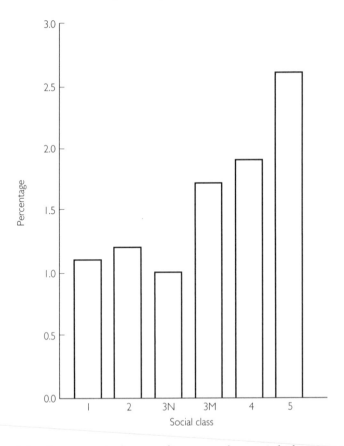

Figure 6.5   Pneumonia by age five years by social class, Great Britain, 1975. (Source [21] p. 93)

Table 6.5 Admission with clinically suspected bronchiolitis and deprivation. (Source [43])

Deprivation level of area of residence	Intervention group (n = 127)	Controls (n = 612)	Odds ratio (OR)
I	11	101	1.00
II	17	95	1.64
III	41	217	1.39
IV	39	127	2.82
V	19	72	2.42

Chi-squared for linear trend 8.869, $P = 0.0029$.

social class children in the 1946 Cohort and they tended to be affected at earlier ages than their more advantaged peers; wheezing, bronchitis and pneumonia were all more common in lower social class children in the 1970 Cohort, though the authors note that the social class differences disappeared after standardisation for other factors such as maternal smoking (*see* Part Three – The causal debate).[39,40] Figure 6.5 shows the marked social class gradient in pneumonia before the age of five years in the children of the 1970 Cohort.

Other UK studies from the 1950s and 1960s, reviewed by Colley, confirm a social class gradient in lower and upper respiratory infections in childhood, and lower SES has been identified as an independent risk factor for severe chest illness before the age of two years in US children.[30,41]

Bronchiolitis, a viral lower respiratory tract infection of infancy usually associated with the respiratory syncytial virus (RSV), has been associated with urban living, overcrowding and poor housing conditions.[42] A case–control study of hospital admissions for clinically suspected bronchiolitis during an outbreak in Sheffield (UK) in the winter of 1989–90, demonstrated increased relative odds of admission for children living in deprived areas of the city.[43] For those infants whose condition required medical intervention during their admission, i.e. those who could be assumed to have a more severe illness, the relative odds were also significantly increased for infants living in deprived areas (*see* Table 6.5).

Despite effective immunisation, pertussis remains prevalent in some communities. An ecological study from Denver, Colorado reported higher age-adjusted rates of pertussis infection in areas with higher proportions of residents with incomes below the poverty level.[44] TB, which is resurgent in less developed (*see* Chapter 5) and developed countries, is closely linked with poverty and overcrowding.[45] The association between socio-economic status and childhood respiratory and other infections is well summarised by Reading.[46]

The evidence related to asthma and recurrent wheezing is less clear. A higher risk of asthma associated with lower SES has been suggested by a few studies.[47,48] However, allergic conditions generally have been shown to have a reverse class gradient in children and young adults and a clear social gradient in asthma is not established.[49] The risk of hospital admission for asthma is increased for children from areas with high poverty levels and there is some evidence that asthma severity may be greater in children from lower SES homes.[8,30,47,48] Children of lower SES families are at higher risk of less clearly defined respiratory conditions and symptoms, such as persistent cough: Colley and Reid reported a prevalence of chronic cough in urban six to ten year olds of 20% in social classes IV and V compared to 10% in social classes I and II.[50] Children in the lower social classes from the 1970 UK National Cohort had a higher prevalence of regular coughing at the age of ten years. In young adults of both sexes, followed as part of the 1958 UK National Cohort, there was a clear social class gradient for respiratory symptoms though not for asthma and wheezy bronchitis.[21,50] Damp housing, especially when associated with fungal mould, has been shown to be linked with increased reporting of respiratory and other symptoms, and cold houses with a twofold increase in respiratory illness among Bengalis living in East London.[51,52]

Next to the respiratory tract, the gastrointestinal tract in infancy and childhood is the most vulnerable to infection. Vomiting and diarrhoea are very frequent in childhood and many such symptoms are managed without medical intervention. As discussed in Chapters 4 and 5, gastroenteritis was a major cause of childhood mortality and morbidity in developed countries prior to improvements in living standards and sanitation, and is still a major cause in less developed countries. There is surprisingly little information on the relationship between gastroenteritis and social factors; what evidence is available indicates a strong class gradient in hospital admission for gastroenteritis.[29,53] Poor children with appendicitis are more likely to experience appendiceal perforation and peritonitis than their non-poor peers.[30]

Information relating medically defined disability in childhood and SES is limited, though there are considerable self-reported disability and incapacity data (*see* below). A retrospective population-based survey of all cases of cerebral palsy born to residents in the Eastern Health Board area of the Republic of Ireland between 1976 and 1981 demonstrated a clear social class gradient in the overall prevalence of cerebral palsy, which was particularly evident in the individual syndromes of hemiplegia and diplegia (Figure 6.6).[54] Prevalence of cerebral palsy

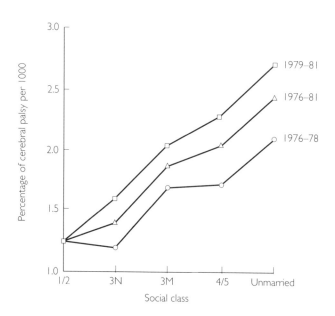

Figure 6.6   Prevalence (per 1000 births) of cerebral palsy by social class among births in the Eastern Health Board of the Republic of Ireland, 1976–78, 1976–81 and 1979–81. (Source [54] p. 193)

severe enough to prevent walking by the child's fourth birthday increased from 0.5/1000 births in social classes I and II to 1.7/1000 in the unmarried group. A retrospective survey in Malta reported a marked social gradient in cerebral palsy.[55] Unpublished data from an ongoing study of childhood disability, using data from all births in the relatively affluent English area of West Sussex between 1975 and 1994, show a social gradient for all types of cerebral palsy but, unlike the Irish data, fail to show any social gradient in severity (Sundrum – personal communication).

Dowding and Barry review other studies relating cerebral palsy to social class and conclude that most are inconclusive or reach inappropriate conclusions owing to problems of method, particularly the failure to estimate prevalence based on a defined population.[54] Townsend, in his study of poverty in the UK in the 1960s, used strict criteria of children with a handicap (including the immobile; those with a 'marked disablement condition'; those attending a special school or training centre) and, though numbers were small, demonstrated an association between living in poverty and having a child with a severe handicap.[56] It was not possible to say from the study whether the association was due to the increased financial penalties of having a child with a handicap, or whether poverty itself had a causative role.

Starfield and Budetti, and Jolly, conclude that poor children are more likely to suffer sequelae of acute illnesses, and chronic diseases are more likely to have a worse impact. For example, poor American children with diabetes are reported to have twice the hospitalisation rate of their more prosperous peers.[57,30]

Iron-deficiency anaemia in early childhood is strongly associated with low SES: a series of UK studies have confirmed this association and US and Russian studies reach the same conclusion.[8,58,59] Children in some ethnic minority groups are particularly vulnerable to iron deficiency (see also Chapter 7): in some groups this seems to be related to dietary practices but much of the effect is related to the poorer socio-economic circumstances of this group of children.[59,60] Iron-deficiency anaemia has been shown to adversely affect psychomotor development and to render children more vulnerable to infection.[61] Other nutritional deficiencies, such as suboptimal levels of vitamins A and E, have been associated with low income.[62]

Children from lower SES homes are known to have an increased risk of a range of other medically defined conditions: squint, children medically defined as 'clumsy', dental caries, lead poisoning alone and in combination with iron-deficiency anaemia, and behavioural problems including soiling and bedwetting (*see* p. 163).[8,57,50,63,64] Otitis media and associated permanent and transient hearing loss have serious educational consequences and have been shown to be more common in disadvantaged children.[65]

Studies from various countries have shown an increased risk of hospital admission among children from disadvantaged homes.[57] Hospital admission has been criticised as a measure of morbidity as the reasons for hospital admission may be related more to variables other than the child's illness, such as the admitting professional's perception of parental coping capacity.[66] Evidence from a case-control study in Sheffield of children experiencing multiple admissions before the age of three years suggests that the increased risk of admission remains even for those children admitted for significant pathologies.[67]

Parent-reported morbidity

The trend to increased use of parent- or self-reported morbidity in studies of childhood ill health was considered in Chapter 3, p. 53. As discussed, these measures have been criticised on the grounds of differential perceptions of illness between social groups, limiting their use as measures of social inequality in child health.[68] Despite these methodological objections, parent-reported morbidity in various age groups studied in the UK and the USA shows a clear gradient by socio-economic status.

Data from the UK General Household Survey (GHS) (1985–89), analysed by Judge and Benzeval and reported by Kumar, are shown in Table 6.6.[5]

For boys, the ratio of social class V/I is 1.46 for chronic illness and 1.73 for limiting illness; for girls, the ratios are 1.17 and 1.85 respectively. Data from the 1991 GHS show that children (male and female) aged 0–19 years from manual

Table 6.6   Childhood morbidity (parent-reported) 0–15 years in Great Britain, 1985–89. (Source [5] p. 109)

Social class	Males (n = 13 949)			Females (n = 13 499)		
	Chronic	Limiting	Acute	Chronic	Limiting	Acute
	%	%	%	%	%	%
I	14.7	5.5	10.9	11.8	3.4	14.4
II	15.5	6.3	11.4	13.7	5.0	11.6
III non-manual	17.4	6.4	13.0	13.0	5.0	13.2
III manual	17.4	7.4	12.0	13.8	5.8	12.4
IV	19.3	9.5	13.3	14.5	5.4	11.1
V	21.4	9.5	13.3	13.8	6.3	12.4
Ratio V/I	1.46	1.73	1.22	1.17	1.85	0.86
All persons	17.2	7.4	12.2	13.4	5.2	12.2

workers' families were reported to have higher rates of limiting long-standing illness than those from non-manual workers' families, with a range from 4.4% in the families of inter-mediate/junior non-manual workers to 7.0% in the families of semi-skilled manual workers.[21] Table 6.7 shows the results of a re-analysis by Judge and Benzeval of data from a survey of living standards of Londoners conducted in 1985–86.[5,69]

These data show a consistent increase in children whose health is reported to be fair/poor with increasing deprivation level. Townsend's survey collected data on the components of what he defines as material and social deprivation (*see* Chapter 2), for example housing deprivation, dietary deprivation and clothing deprivation.

Multivariate analysis of the data by Judge and Benzeval allows them to estimate the variance in reported fair/poor health accounted for by the individual components of deprivation: the worst housing deprivation accounted for 0.27 of the variance; maximum score on all elements of material deprivation accounted for 0.71 of the variance; maximum score on all adverse circumstances (social as well as material deprivation) accounted for 0.96 of the variance.[5]

Table 6.7   Deprivation and child health in London, 1985–86. (Source [5] p. 140)

Individual	Deprivation categories				n =
	1 (least deprived)	2	3	4 (most deprived)	
	%	%	%	%	
Good	95.9	92.4	81.9	64.9	782
Fair/poor	4.1	7.6	18.1	35.1	148
n =	147	330	248	205	930

The same gradient in reported morbidity has been noted in US studies: children from low income families are reported to have 30% more days when their activity is restricted and 40% more days lost from school due to illness.[30] Three to six times the proportion of poor children are reported by their teachers to be in fair or poor health and three times as many have a condition reported by the teachers to limit schoolwork or play.[30]

A small number of studies explore the relationship between reported morbidity in children and specific aspects of the home environment. Damp housing is reported to be associated with increased levels of reported respiratory and other symptoms.[51] A US study suggests that reported morbidity is higher in homeless than in housed children.[70]

The social gradient in reported long-standing limiting illness seems to become less marked in young adults, though the gradient again becomes more marked after this age.[49,71]

Birth weight and growth

Low birth weight

In developed as in developing countries (*see* Chapter 5), low birth weight (LBW) is strongly correlated with measures of SES. Data from Scotland in 1978 show that 5.3% of babies born to wives of professional men weighed less than 2.5 kg compared with 9.8% of babies born to wives of unskilled men.[72] More recent UK studies, using measures of area deprivation (*see* Chapter 1), show a marked trend in LBW from least deprived to most deprived.[73,74]

Similar gradients related to measures of SES are reported from Spain, Sweden and the USA.[8,75,76] LBW rates are twice as high in American blacks as in American whites and almost three times higher in babies of Australian Aboriginal mothers than in those of Australian white mothers.[77] As will be discussed in Chapter 7, these differences are at least in part a reflection of socio-economic differences.

LBW incorporates two broad groups of babies: those born preterm and those who are small for their gestational age (SGA). Low SES appears to increase the risk of both preterm and SGA birth.[8,76] Though not a measure of morbidity, LBW is the most powerful determinant of perinatal survival.[78] It is closely correlated with ill health in the neonatal period as well as death and with hospital admission before the age of two years.[67,79] LBW influences adult height attained and has been linked to premature death from coronary artery disease.[49,80]

Although low birth weight has been the main research focus, mean birthweight of whole populations and population subgroups is arguably a more valuable measure of the health status. Along with rates of fetal loss, it is a summary measure of the reproductive efficiency of a population. Over the ten years 1985–94, the mean birth weight of babies born in Sheffield, UK increased by 34 g mainly due to an increase in births weighing >3500 g and a corresponding decrease in those born between 3000 and 3499 g.[81] The increase was the same in all social groups, however there was a consistent difference in mean birth weight of around 170 g between the most and the least disadvantaged deciles of the population across all the years studied. Figure 6.7 shows the social gradient in mean birth weight for the West Midlands Health Region of England in the years 1991–93. The difference between the most and least disadvantaged deciles was 220 g. In this study, more than 30% of the births <2500 g were statistically 'attributable' to social inequality.[82] The Sheffield study[81] explored social differences in

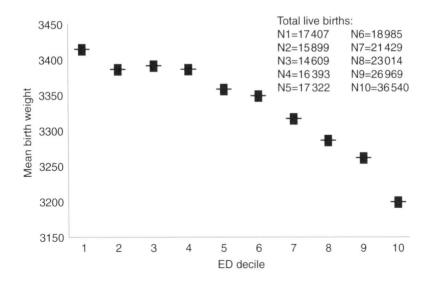

Figure 6.7   Mean birth weight for all live births by Enumeration District (ED) decile. Ranked by Townsend Deprivation Index: West Midlands Health Region, 1991–93.

birth weight at the other end of the range, babies born >3500 g: social inequality accounted for 9.6% of births over the ten years which fell below this optimal level.

A similar social gradient in mean birth weight was noted in Goteborg, Sweden;[83] however, mean birth weights in the Swedish city were 200 g higher than in Sheffield and the West Midlands, resulting in a higher proportion of infants in the optimal birth weight group and fewer low birth weight babies. The most disadvantaged group in Goteborg, 1982–86, had a mean birth weight (3390 g) greater than that for all Sheffield births, 1990–94 (3310 g).

A study comparing mean birth weight by educational group in the Czech Republic and Sweden[84] found a similar difference between mean birth weights in the two countries (Czech Republic, 3310 g; Sweden, 3522 g) as seen between the UK studies and Goteborg. Difference in mean birth weight for infants of mothers with primary and university education was 197 g (95% CI, 190 205) in the Czech Republic and 136 g (95% CI, 128 144) in Sweden. The study also reported that mean birth weight in the Czech Republic fell 31 g between 1989 and 1991, associated with a widening of social differences and more worsening in the lower socio-economic groups.

Growth

Differences in adult height attained related to SES are well recognised and have been noted for many years.[85,86] These differences are present in developing (*see* Chapter 5) and developed countries and, though they decreased in the 1950s in Sweden, they reasserted themselves in the 1960s, and for the UK Carr-Hill found 'no discernible narrowing either of the overall distribution or of the gap between social classes' between 1940 and 1980.[85,87] RGSC I and II 15-year-old Newcastle children studied in the 1960s were on average 4.5 cm taller than RGSC IV and V children.[88] Data from the 1958 UK National Cohort Study (NCDS), analysed by Lasker and Mascie-Taylor, show mean heights at 16 years of 172.5 cm for RGSC I boys and 163.1 cm for RGSC I girls compared with 167.8 for RGSC V boys and 159.0 for RGSC V girls.[89] Using data from the same cohort, Davie and co-workers showed that at the extremes of advantage and disadvantage, the difference in average height of the children at the age of seven years was as great as 13.8 cm.[63] More recent data from the Wessex (UK) Growth Study[90] showed that very short normal children were significantly more likely to be from low socio-economic status households than their age- and sex-matched controls.

Similar differences have been reported from countries as diverse as Poland and Sweden.[91,92] The differences between socio-economic groups appear to become established before the age of seven years, varying little after that time, and factors present at birth, such as mid-parental height and birth weight, exert a strong influence on eventual height attained.[49,89]

Small stature, like LBW, is not an illness. However, there is considerable evidence that it is correlated with adverse outcomes in adult life: small stature has been linked to an increased risk of coronary artery disease and of mortality from obstructive lung diseases.[80,93,94] Maternal height has a strong influence on pregnancy outcome.[72]

Other parameters related to health

There are other aspects of children's life experience which are closely related to health. These have been characterised as part of the 'new' morbidity and are principally related to emotional and family difficulties.[95] They can be broadly divided into life events which are associated with adverse health outcomes and health-related problems which frequently present to the caring agencies. Both are closely linked with socio-economic circumstances.

Life events associated with adverse child health outcomes

Divorce and marital conflict

Breakdown of their parents' marriage/relationship is one of the most traumatic events in the life of a child, though the extent of the effects is disputed.[96] Divorce and separation are now frequent events in the lives of many children in developed countries. Studies in Sweden suggest that families in poor socio-economic circumstances are more vulnerable to family breakdown.[97] This finding is supported by evidence that marital conflict is increased and parenting impaired by acute and chronic socio-economic adversity.[98]

Lone parenthood

Associated with the increased tendency for relationships to break down is the trend in lone parenthood. Throughout most of the developed world and particularly the UK, the USA and the Nordic countries over the last 20 years, lone parenthood has increased.[96] In the UK between 1981 and 1998, the number of lone-parent families rose from 850 000 to 1.7 million. One fifth of all families with dependent children are now headed by a lone parent and it is estimated that three million children are growing up in these families.[4] As considered in Chapter 2, p. 43, lone parenthood in most countries is closely linked with the experience of relative poverty. Families which experience material and social deprivation are less stable and more vulnerable to breakdown, with the consequence that lone parenthood associated with marriage breakdown in part results from poor socio-economic circumstances.[97,98] Women who have never been married and are unsupported by a partner constitute about a third of lone parents in the UK and the USA. These women are often young and have been held responsible for the development of a so-called 'underclass' (*see* also Chapter 10).[99] Young women from families in poor socio-economic circumstances are at greatly increased risk of becoming unsupported lone parents.[4,6]

Teenage pregnancy

An associated phenomenon is teenage pregnancy, which has been related to adverse outcomes for both the infant and the mother. A study from Scotland illustrates how closely this phenomenon is linked with material deprivation: girls under 16 years of age from deprived areas were three times more likely to become pregnant than their more privileged peers but less likely to have the pregnancy terminated.[100] It has been suggested that teenagers become pregnant in order to give them an advantage in the queue for social housing. However, evidence from a number of studies suggests that lack of employment prospects contributes to the decision of teenage girls to continue with the pregnancy – in other words, becoming a mother is a 'career' choice for girls with no qualifications and no prospects of regular work.[101]

Data from the USA[102] and Canada[14] show that teenage pregnancy is closely linked to poverty: 11% of poor US teenage girls have an out-of-wedlock birth compared with 3.6% of non-poor; 18% of teenage women (16–19) from low income families in Ontario, Canada had been pregnant in the five years up to 1990 compared with 4% in high income families.

While teenage pregnancy is undoubtedly an adverse health outcome for many young women and their children, the associated moral panic[99] is misguided: as shown, in Figure 6.8, births to teenage mothers have fallen in all European countries though it is notable that the rate of fall in the UK has been slower than comparable countries.[4]

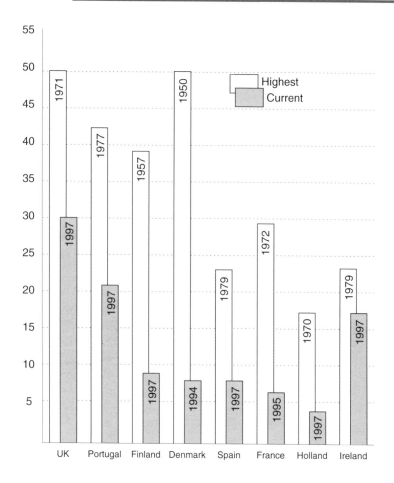

Figure 6.8 Comparative trends in births (per 1000) to women aged 15–19: selected European countries. (Source [4] p. 233)

Educational underachievement and youth unemployment

Educational underachievement and youth unemployment are closely linked and are both strongly correlated with poor socio-economic circumstances.[5] Evidence from the UK National Child Development Study showed a clear link between poor attainment in reading at ages seven and 11 and disadvantage.[103] More recent evidence confirms that poor educational attainment and socio-economic status are closely linked: in the UK, over 75%

of the between-school variance in the proportion of pupils achieving five or more grades, A to C, at GCSE is explained by reference to the socio-economic backgrounds of the pupils;[104] Canadian data demonstrate a clear negative gradient in maths scores, by income, among children aged 4–11 years from two-parent families.[105] There is also evidence that, against a background of increased national levels of educational attainment, inner-city schools in some particularly deprived areas of the UK have shown no increase or an actual decline.[5] Grade repetition, expulsion and suspension and high school drop-out rates are all significantly higher in poor US children than their non-poor peers.[102] School truancy rates are also closely linked to material and social deprivation.[106] Similar findings have been reported from the USA; Wolfe states:

> *Children in poor families are three times more likely to drop out of high school than are children in more prosperous families, and each year a child lives in poverty reduces his or her probability of graduation by nearly 1%.*[107]

Youth unemployment in developed countries has risen in line with the general rise in unemployment in the 1980s. Since the war, young people have become more vulnerable to unemployment, and unemployment rates amongst 16–19 year-olds and young adults (20–24 years) have been particularly high in the 1980s and 1990s.[4] Between winter 1997–98 and winter 1998–99, the unemployment rate (using the International Labour Organisation definition) among 16–17 year-olds increased from 19.8% to 20.8% despite a reduction in the overall unemployment rate.[4] Unemployment differentially affects young people from low income families: family poverty and disadvantage are the major determinants of non-participation in education or work post-16 years in the UK;[4] 15.9% of poor US 24 year-olds are economically inactive compared with 8.3% of non-poor;[102] among 16–19 year-olds in Canada, there is a steep negative gradient in non-participation from 16% in families with incomes <C$20 000 to 4% in families with incomes ≥C$80 000.[105]

Table 6.8   Risk of admission to care by socio-demographic factors. (Source [87] p. 354)

Child 'A'	Child 'B'
Aged 5–9	Aged 5–9
No state benefit	Household head receives state benefit
2-parent family	Single adult household
≤3 children	≥4 children
Owner-occupied house	Private rented home
More rooms than people	1+ persons per room

Probability of child going into care	
Child 'A'	Child 'B'
1:7000	1:10

Admission into care

Admission of a child into care is a traumatic event which can have serious health, particularly mental health, consequences for the child and the family. Table 6.8, derived from a case–control study of children admitted to local authority care in the UK, shows the striking difference in risk of admission to care between child 'A' with few adverse material and family factors and child 'B' with a range of adverse material and family factors.[108] The results shown in Table 6.8 indicate that, as with other adverse life events, poor socio-economic circumstances are associated with an increased risk of admission into care.

Health problems related to emotional and family disturbance

Parenting is the common factor by which many of the health problems related to emotional and family disturbance are thought to be mediated.[109] However, parenting is not simply a function of the competence or psychological make-up of the individual parent, but it takes place within a social context. Socio-economic disadvantage, acting through increased marital conflict, poorer material environments and higher levels of parental mental health and chronic stress, adversely affects child rearing.[98] As with many of the adverse health outcomes considered in this chapter, there is a finely graded social patterning of many of the factors which affect child rearing: for example, the proportion of children living with a parent showing frequent signs of depression in the 1994–95 Canadian National Population Health Survey[105] varied from 22% in the lowest income group to 6% in the highest group. The gradient for children living with parents experiencing high levels of chronic stress was in the same direction, from 12.5% in the lowest income group to 3.5% in the highest.

Child abuse and neglect

Child abuse and neglect (CA&N), including child sexual abuse (CSA), has been the focus of increasing interest and concern among child care professionals and governments in developed countries in recent years. Much research has concentrated on family pathology. However, increasing evidence is emerging for the link between poor socio-economic circumstances and CA&N. This evidence, summarised by Baldwin and Spencer, comes mainly from studies in the UK and the USA.[110] Much of the evidence is based on case identification through available abuse registers, which have been criticised as being part of a mechanism of social control with a greater chance of detection and registration in poor families.[111] In other words there is a built-in reporting bias.[112] However, the extent and consistency of the links found when they have been sought are compelling. Some of the most convincing evidence comes from a study in the USA which shows a consistent link between low family income and registration across all categories of CA&N.[113]

Failure to thrive and childhood obesity

Failure to thrive (FTT) in infancy is frequently linked to CA&N though it is now clear that many cases are not directly related to abuse or neglect.[114] Whether or not non-organic FTT is abusive in origin, it is clear that it is closely correlated with poor socio-economic circumstances; studies in Newcastle, UK (Wright – personal communication) and in the USA show consistent links with poverty and low SES.[114] Frank and Zeisel state:

> *Poverty is the most important single social risk factor for failure to thrive because of the close association between poverty and childhood malnutrition. Although failure to thrive may occur in children of all social classes, most clinical cases come from low-income families.* ([114] p. 1194)

At the other end of the spectrum of malnutrition, obesity is linked with diabetes, hypertension and coronary artery disease.[115] Childhood obesity seems to be increasing among UK children.[5] There is conflicting evidence concerning the relationship between socio-economic status and childhood obesity, but there is a strong consistent relationship between low socio-economic status in early life and increased adult obesity.[116]

Behavioural and mental health problems

Behavioural and mental health problems in childhood are common.[21] A Disability Survey by the UK Office of Populations, Censuses and Surveys (OPCS) between 1985 and 1988 identified behavioural problems as the main category of functional disability at all ages of childhood, with prevalences of 13/1000 at 0–4 years, 23/1000 at 5–9 years and 25/1000 at 10–15 years.[117] Behavioural and emotional problems in childhood are more commonly reported in children of families with lower SES: data from the 1970 UK National Birth Cohort show that among the worst 10% of children on a behavioural continuum, RGSC V children had higher prevalences at the age of ten in hyperactivity, conduct disorder and anxiety.[21]

Recent evidence from Canada[105] and the UK[118] demonstrates a steep negative gradient in a range of behaviour problems by income (see Figure 6.9). Enuresis, one of the most common behavioural and developmental problems of childhood, is linked with low socio-economic status.[119] Attention deficit hyperactivity disorder (ADHD), an increasingly recognised and diagnosed problem of childhood, has been linked to low income,[120] as have DSM-III-R psychiatric disorders.[121] Parker

DSM IV

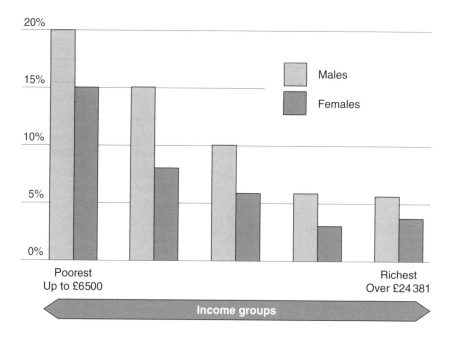

Figure 6.9   Difficult children and income: percentage of children aged 4–15 with emotional/behavioural difficulties. (Source [118])

and co-workers characterised the process by which poor children suffer a higher prevalence of behavioural and developmental problems as 'double jeopardy': first, poor children are more likely to be exposed to risk factors which are positively correlated with adverse outcomes, and second, the effects of these risk factors tend to be greater than they are for non-poor children.[122] One of these major risk factors is maternal depression, which is closely correlated with SES.[105] Maternal depression has been linked with, among others, FTT in infancy, sleep problems, childhood depression and withdrawn and defiant behaviour in adolescence.[122,123]

Gender inequalities and child health in developed countries

The phenomenon of 'hidden' poverty, particularly affecting women and children, related to the maldistribution of family resources was considered in Chapter 1. There are few data relating directly to the effects of hidden poverty on the health of the woman or her children. As Oakley and co-workers point out, 'most analyses of class and health have focused narrowly on death as a health outcome and on male experience'.[124] Women are often left out of the analysis or it is assumed that social class affects women's health in the same way as it does for men.[125]

Trends in social inequalities in infant and childhood health

The data presented above demonstrate with remarkable consistency the relationship between socio-economic factors measured in various ways and death and ill health in infancy and childhood in developed countries, all of which have experienced precipitous falls in mortality rates during the last 100 years. Figure 6.2 indicates that the UK social class gradient has been maintained throughout much of the general fall in IMR. An exception to this general trend appeared to be the PNMR for England and Wales in the 1970s when the differential between the classes apparently narrowed.[126] Various explanations were advanced for this narrowing, including the decreasing proportion of the population in RGSC V. However, re-analysis of the data by Pamuk, using an index of inequality and including births outside marriage, excluded from the reported OPCS data, demonstrated that the ratio of inequality had remained the same from the 1950s onwards (Figure 6.10).[127]

Table 6.9 shows that for births within marriage (OPCS data) the ratio RGSC V:RGSC I for IMR for England and Wales rose from 1.8 in 1978–79 to 2.0 in 1990. For perinatal deaths, the ratio fell from 1.71 to 1.59 between 1978 and 1987 and for neonatal deaths rose from 1.49 to 1.51.

When infant deaths among those births within, and jointly registered outside, marriage are considered, the ratio of RGSC V:I between 1987 and 1988 and 1988 and 1989 rose from 1.73 to 1.89.[5] Mortality trends examined for the Northern Health

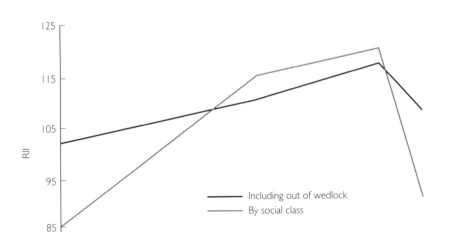

Figure 6.10   Relative index of inequality in post-neonatal mortality, 1920–80, by social class, excluding those infants born outside marriage, compared with indices when out-of-wedlock infants are included. The relative index of inequality (RII) is calculated from the difference between extreme social groups so that a 2.1 difference ≡ an RII of 100. (Source [127])

Region of England using area deprivation indices (*see* Chapter 1 for discussion of area deprivation indices) show that for the most deprived fifth of the electoral wards in the region, the age-standardised mortality in 0–14 year-olds rose from 116 in 1981–83 to 130 in 1989–91 compared with a slight fall from 80 to 79 in the least deprived areas.[128] The decline in death rates from injury and poisoning among children aged 0–15 years in England and Wales between 1979–83 and 1989–92 was 2% for children in social class V compared with 32% for those in social class I, with the result that the injury death rate for social class V children was five times that of social class I children in the four-year period, 1989–92.[129]

In the USA, the ratio of non-white to white infants born with a birth weight of less than 2.5 kg is reported to have increased from 1975 to the mid-1980s, while the IMR differential

Table 6.9 Stillbirths and infant deaths by father's social class (defined by occupation at death registration) for the period 1978–90, England and Wales (for births within marriage only). (Source [5] p. 102)

Social class	1990					1978–87			
	Still-birth	Perinatal death	Neonatal death	Post-neonatal death	Infant death	Perinatal death		Neonatal death	
						1978	1987	1978	1987
All	4.3	7.4	4.1	2.6	6.7	14.8	8.2	8.3	4.7
I–V	4.3	7.4	4.0	2.5	6.5	–	–	–	–
I	3.6	6.6	3.6	2.0	5.6	11.9	6.8	6.8	3.9
II	3.4	6.0	3.3	2.0	5.3	12.3	7.0	7.0	4.1
IIIN	4.1	7.1	4.0	2.3	6.4	13.9	7.8	7.9	4.4
IIIM	4.4	7.6	4.1	2.4	6.5	15.1	8.1	8.1	4.5
IV	5.7	9.5	4.8	3.5	8.3	16.7	9.9	9.3	5.6
V	5.6	9.6	5.8	5.4	11.2	20.3	10.8	10.1	5.9
Other	4.9	9.1	5.9	4.6	10.5	20.4	9.9	14.4	6.8
Ratio V/I	1.56	1.45	1.61	2.7	2.0	1.71	1.59	1.49	1.51

between the groups for the same period remained constant.[130] The former Communist bloc countries have witnessed an actual decline in child health in the ten years following the collapse of the USSR and its European satellite states. Diphtheria and tuberculosis have increased dramatically among the poor in Russia as have suicide rates among young people in Russia and the Czech Republic.[131] The mean birth weight in the Czech Republic decreased significantly between 1989 and 1991 as a result of more rapid worsening in the lower socio-economic groups.[84] By contrast, Italian data comparing 1975 and 1980–83 show a declining trend from 2.6 to 1.8 in the IMR between infants born to mothers with no or primary-only education and mothers with a college education.[11] In Sweden, over the last century, differences in mortality between infants of married and unmarried mothers have virtually disappeared although socio-economic differentials persist, albeit at a low level.[25] Infant mortality differentials between Spanish regions which were based on socio-economic factors have reduced between 1975–78 and 1983–86.[25]

Social groups are not static: they undergo change over time in response to economic and demographic changes in populations. Equally, diseases and their social distribution can change with potential effects on health inequalities; the best-known example of this process is coronary artery disease, which has changed from a disease of 'affluence' affecting mainly men in developed countries to a disease of lower class men and women living in affluent societies.[132] Deaths and paralysis associated with poliomyelitis showed an unexpected class gradient from high in higher social groups to low in lower social groups in the major epidemics of the 1930s and early 1950s; later the class gradient reversed.[78] It appeared that the virus was acquired through 'good living'. However, the explanation lay in the overcrowded social conditions of poor children who acquired the virus early in infancy when still protected by passive immunity from their mothers; children from more affluent homes who had not had asymptomatic infections in early infancy were highly susceptible to infection at a slightly older age. The class gradient reversed as a result of differential uptake of immunisation in higher class children.

Health inequalities and relative poverty

The data presented in this chapter from various developed countries show a consistent positive correlation of adverse health outcomes, including death and a range of illnesses, parent-reported morbidity and factors associated with poor health, and low SES measured in a variety of ways. As considered in Chapter 1, the definition of 'relative' poverty is problematic and different countries use different measures to define a poverty line.

How do the various measures of SES used in the studies described above relate to the concept of relative poverty? In the case of the US data which refer directly to the 'poor', the measure is based on the official US poverty lines (*see* Chapter 1). In some US data, race is a proxy for economic factors and the non-white groups in the USA experience much higher levels of poverty (*see* Chapter 2 for the extent of poverty and Chapter 7 for a discussion of the relationship between race, poverty and health). Data based on occupational class, usually of the male head of the household, such as the RGSC classification, present more problems. However, there is consistent evidence from the UK of a positive association between low income and the lower social classes using the RGSC classification.[56] For unoccupied mothers, the association with low income is even closer.[33]

Area and regional measures such as deprivation indices are based on income proxies such as unemployment levels, housing tenure and car ownership in the UK (*see* Chapter 1), derived from Census data. These have been shown to correlate closely with the experience of those living in these areas of either privilege or relative poverty. The description of regions of countries as 'rich' or 'poor' is based on the GNP of the region or its relative level of industrialisation, as in the case of the republics of former Yugoslavia or the regions of Italy. These descriptions strongly correlate not only with GNP or level of industrialisation but also with the actual living standards of the people living in them.

Thus, though not precise measures of relative poverty, the measures of SES reflect the experience of relative poverty of individual families or geographically defined populations.

Summary

1   There is a consistent positive correlation between low SES and adverse late pregnancy and child health outcomes in developed countries which holds for mortality at all ages and for measures of medically defined morbidity and parent-reported morbidity.

2   This correlation holds good in all developed countries in which it has been sought, though it is weaker in those such as Sweden where socio-economic differences are less marked.

3   There is a consistent positive correlation in developed countries between low SES and the 'new' morbidity related to family and emotional disturbance.

4   There is a consistent positive correlation in developed countries between low SES and educational attainment and life events which can adversely affect health.

5   In some countries, notably the UK and the USA, there is evidence that, despite the overall fall in infant mortality rates, there is no reduction in the differential in IMRs between the most and the least privileged groups and there is tentative evidence that the gap is widening. Over the last decade, in the former Communist bloc countries of Eastern and Central Europe there has been a general decline in child health, mainly affecting those who have been impoverished as a consequence of profound social and economic changes.

References

1   Kohler L (1991) Infant mortality – the Swedish experience. *Annu. Rev. Public Health.* **12**:177–93.

2   McKeown T (1976) *The Role of Medicine: Dream, Mirage or Nemesis?* The Nuffield Hospitals Trust, London.

3   Rose G (1991) *The Strategy of Preventative Medicine.* Oxford University Press, Oxford.

4   NCH Action for Children (1999) *Factfile 2000: Facts and Figures on Issues Facing Britain's Children.* NCH Action for Children, London.

5   Kumar V (1993) *Poverty and Inequality in the UK: The Effects on Children.* National Children's Bureau, London.

6   Danziger S and Stern J (1990) *The causes and consequences of child poverty in the United States.* Innocenti Occasional Papers, No. 10, Unicef International Child Development Centre, Florence, Italy.

7   Fingerhut LA, Wilson RW and Feldman JJ (1980) Health and disease in the United States. *Annu. Rev. Public Health.* 1:1–36.

8   Wise P and Meyers A (1988) Poverty and child health. *Paediatr. Clin. North Am.* 35:1169–86.

9   Saraceno C (1990) *Child poverty and deprivation in Italy: 1950 to present.* Innocenti Occasional Papers, No. 6, Unicef International Child Development Centre, Florence, Italy.

10   Cornia GA (1990) *Child poverty and deprivation in industrialized countries: recent trends and policy options.* Innocenti Occasional Papers, No. 2, Unicef International Child Development Centre, Florence, Italy.

11   Parazzini F (1992) Social class differences in infant mortality rate [letter]. *BMJ.* 305:1228.

12   United Nations (1992) *Levels and Trends of Mortality since 1950.* United Nations, New York.

13   Antonovsky A and Bernstein J (1977) Social class and infant mortality. *Soc. Sci. Med.* 11:453–70.

14   Ross DP, Scott K and Kelly M (1996) *Child Poverty: What Are The Consequences?* Centre for International Statistics, Canadian Council on Social Development, Ottawa, Canada.

15   Elmen H (1993) Infant mortality – social inequality in a Swedish city. *Eur. J. Public Health.* 3:237–41.

16   Mastilica M (1990) Health and social inequality in Yugoslavia. *Soc. Sci. Med.* **31**:405–12.

17   Mivev D, Dermendjieva B and Mileva N (1990) The Bulgarian country profile: the dynamics of some health inequalities. *Soc. Sci. Med.* **31**:837–46.

18   Orosz E (1990) The Hungarian country profile: inequalities in health and healthcare in Hungary. *Soc. Sci. Med.* **31**: 847–57.

19   Wnuk-Lipinski E (1990) The Polish country profile: economic crisis and inequalities in health. *Soc. Sci. Med.* **31**:859–66.

20   Wnuk-Lipinski E and Illsley R (1990) International comparative analysis: main findings and conclusions. *Soc. Sci. Med.* **31**:879–89.

21   Woodroffe C, Glickman M, Barker M *et al.* (1993) *Children, Teenagers and Health: The Key Data.* Open University Press, Milton Keynes.

22   Tzoumaka-Bakoula C, Lekea-Karanika V, Matsaniotis NS *et al.* (1989) Are there gaps in the provision of perinatal care in Greece? *J. Epidemiol. Community Health.* **43**:319–23.

23   Bambang S, Spencer NJ, Logan S *et al.* (2000). Cause-specific perinatal death rates, birth weight and deprivation in the West Midlands, 1985–94. *Child: care, health and development.* **26**:73–82.

24   Leon DA (1991) Influence of birth weight on differences in infant mortality by social class and legitimacy. *BMJ.* **303**: 964–7.

25   Drever F and Whitehead M (1997) *Health Inequalities: Decennial Supplement (DS No. 15).* The Stationery Office, London.

26   Spencer NJ and Logan S (2000) Sudden unexpected death in infancy and socio-economic status: a systematic review. *Paediatr. Perinat. Epidemiol.* In press.

27 Department of Health (1996) *Confidential Enquiry into Stillbirths and Deaths in Infancy: 3rd Annual Report (1st January–31st December, 1994)*. DoH, London.

28 Dalviet AK, Irgens LM, Oyen N *et al.* (1998) Socio-demographic risk factors for sudden infant death syndrome: association with other risk factors. *Acta Paediatr. Scand.* 87:284–90.

29 Towner E, Dowdswell T and Jarvis S (1993) *Reducing Childhood Accidents*. Health Education Authority, London.

30 Starfield B and Budetti PP (1985) Child health status and risk factors. *Health Serv. Res.* 19:817–86.

31 Ostberg V (1997) The social patterning of child mortality: the importance of social class, gender, family structure, immigrant status and population density. *Sociol. Health and Illness.* 19:415–35.

32 Sharples PM, Storey A, Aynsley-Green A *et al.* (1990) Causes of fatal childhood accidents involving head injury in Northern region, 1979–1986. *BMJ.* 301:1193–7.

33 Judge K and Benzeval M (1993) Health inequalities: new concerns about the children of single mothers. *BMJ.* 306: 677–80.

34 Takala AK and Clements DA (1992) Socio-economic risk factors for invasive *Haemophilus influenzae* type b disease. *J. Infect. Dis.* 165(1):S11–S15.

35 Gordis L, Lilienfield A and Rodriguez R (1969) Studies in the epidemiology and preventability of rheumatic fever: socioeconomic factors and the incidence of acute attacks. *J. Chron. Dis.* 21:655–66.

36 Northern Territory Health (1986) *Health Indicators in the Northern Territory*. Northern Territory Health Department, Darwin, Australia.

37 Baker M (1996) Rheumatic fever in New Zealand in the 1990s: still cause for concern. *NZ Public Health Report.* 3:17–19.

38 Golding J (1984) Britain's National Cohort studies. In *Progress in Child Health, Vol. 1* (ed. JA Macfarlane). Churchill Livingstone, Edinburgh.

39 Douglas JWB (1951) Health and survival of infants in different social classes: a national survey. *Lancet.* 2:440–6.

40 Golding J and Butler N (1986) *From Birth to Five.* Pergamon Press, Oxford.

41 Colley JRT (1976) Epidemiology of respiratory disease in childhood. In *Recent Advances in Paediatrics, No. 5* (ed. D Hull). Churchill Livingstone, Edinburgh.

42 Medical Research Council (MRC) Subcommittee on RSV Vaccines (1978) Respiratory syncytial virus infections: admissions to hospital in industrial, urban and rural areas. *BMJ.* 2:796–8.

43 Spencer NJ, Logan S, Scholey S *et al.* (1996) Bronchiolitis and deprivation. *Arch. Dis. Child.* 74:50–2.

44 Seigel C, Davidson A, Kafadar K *et al.* (1997) Geographic analysis of pertussis infection in an urban area: a tool for health service planning. *Am. J. Public Health.* 87:2022–6.

45 Cantwell MF, McKenna MT, McCray E *et al.* (1998) Tuberculosis and race/ethnicity in the United States: the impact of socio-economic status. *Am. J. Resp. Crit. Care Med.* 157:1016–20.

46 Reading R (1997) Social disadvantage and infection in childhood. *Sociol. Health and Illness.* 19:395–414.

47 Schwartz J, Gold D, Dockery D *et al.* (1990) Predictors of asthma and persistent wheeze in a national sample of children in the United States. *Am. Rev. Resp. Dis.* 142:555–62.

48 Wissow LS, Gittelsohn AM, Szklo M *et al.* (1988) Poverty, race and hospitalization for childhood asthma. *Am. J. Public Health.* **78**:777–82.

49 Power C, Manor O and Fox J (1991) *Health and Class: The Early Years.* Chapman and Hall, London.

50 Colley JRT and Reid DD (1970) Urban and social origins of childhood bronchitis in England and Wales. *BMJ.* **2**:213–17.

51 Martin C, Platt SD and Hunt SM (1987) Housing conditions and ill health. *BMJ.* **299**:1547–51.

52 Hyndman SJ (1990) Housing dampness and health among British Bengalis in East London. *Soc. Sci. Med.* **30**:131–41.

53 Ellis ME, Watson B, Mandal B *et al.* (1984) Contemporary gastroenteritis of infancy: clinical features and prehospital management. *BMJ.* **288**:521–3.

54 Dowding WM and Barry C (1990) Cerebral palsy: social class differences in prevalence in relation to birth weight and severity of disability. *J. Epidemiol. Community Health.* **44**: 191–5.

55 Sciberras C and Spencer NJ (1999) Cerebral palsy in Malta, 1981–1991. *Dev. Med. Child Neurol.* **41**:508–11.

56 Townsend P (1979) *Poverty in the United Kingdom.* Penguin, Harmondsworth.

57 Jolly DL (1990) *The Impact of Adversity on Child Health: Poverty and Disadvantage.* Australian College of Paediatrics, Parkville, Victoria.

58 Aukett MA and Wharton BA (1995) Suboptimal nutrition. In *Social Paediatrics* (eds B Lindstrom and NJ Spencer). Oxford University Press, Oxford.

59 Kohlmeier L, Mendez M, Shalnova S *et al.* (1998) Deficient dietary iron intakes among women and children in Russia: evidence from the Russian Longitudinal Monitoring Study. *Am. J. Public Health.* **88**:576–80.

60   James J, Brown J, Douglas M *et al.* (1992) Improving the diet of under-fives in a deprived inner city practice. *Health Trends.* **24**:161–4.

61   Aukett MA, Parks YA and Scott PH (1986) Treatment with iron increases weight gain and psychomotor development. *Arch. Dis. Child.* **61**:849–57.

62   Spannaus-Martin DJ, Cook LR, Tanumihardjo SA *et al.* (1997) Vitamin A and vitamin E statuses of preschool children of socioeconomically disadvantaged families living in the midwestern United States. *Eur. J. Clin. Nutr.* **51**:864–9.

63   Davie R, Butler N and Goldstein H (1972) *From Birth to Seven.* Longmans, London.

64   Carmichael CL, Rugg-Gun AJ and Ferrell RS (1989) The relationship between fluoridation, social class and caries experience in 5-year-old children in Newcastle and Northumberland. *Br. Dent. J.* **167**:57–61.

65   Paradise JL (1980) Otitis media in infants and children. *Paediatr.* **65**:917–43.

66   Rosenburg K (1984) Poverty and the health of children [letter]. *Lancet.* **ii**:814.

67   Spencer NJ, Lewis MA and Logan S (1993) Multiple admission and deprivation. *Arch. Dis. Child.* **68**:760–2.

68   Blane D, Power C and Bartley M (1996) Illness behaviour and the measurement of class differentials in morbidity. *J. Roy. Stat. Soc.* **Series A.** **159**:77–92.

69   Townsend P, Corrigan P and Kowarzik U (1987) *Poverty and Labour in London: Interim Report of the Centenary Survey.* Low Pay Unit, London.

70   Wood DL, Burciaga Valdez R, Hayashi T *et al.* (1990) Health of homeless children and housed, poor children. *Paediatr.* **86**:858–66.

71 West P (1988) Inequality? Social class differences in health in British youth. *Soc. Sci. Med.* **27**:291–6.

72 Macfarlane A and Chambers I (1981) Problems in the interpretation of perinatal mortality statistics. In *Recent Advances in Paediatrics, No. 6* (ed. D Hull). Churchill Livingstone, Edinburgh.

73 Carstairs V and Morris R (1992) *Deprivation and Health in Scotland.* Aberdeen University Press, Aberdeen.

74 Reading R, Openshaw S and Jarvis SN (1990) Measuring child health inequalities using aggregations of enumeration districts. *J. Public Health Med.* **12**:160–7.

75 Armero MJ, Frau MJ and Colomer C (1991) Health indicators for urban areas: geographic variation according to social coherence. *Gaceta Sanitaria* (Spanish). **22**:17–20.

76 Ericson A, Eriksson M, Westerholm P *et al.* (1984) Pregnancy outcome and social indicators in Sweden. *Acta Paediatr. Scand.* **73**:69–74.

77 Seward JF and Stanley FJ (1981) Comparison of births to aboriginal and caucasian mothers in Western Australia. *Med. J. Aust.* **2**:80–4.

78 Susser MW, Watson W and Hopper K (1985) *Sociology in Medicine.* Oxford University Press, New York.

79 Illsley R and Mitchell RG (eds) (1984) *Low Birth Weight: A Medical, Psychological and Social Study.* Wiley, London.

80 Barker DJP (1992) *Fetal and Infant Origins of Adult Disease.* BMJ Publications Group, London.

81 Spencer NJ, Logan S and Gill L (1999) Trends and social patterning of birth weight in Sheffield, 1985–94. *Arch. Dis. Child.* (Fetal and Neonatal Edition). **81**:F138–40.

82 Spencer NJ, Bambang S, Logan S *et al.* (1999) Socioeconomic status and birth weight: comparison of an area-based measure with the Registrar General's social class. *J. Epidemiol. Community Health.* **53**:495–98.

83 Elmen H, Hoglund D, Karlberg P *et al.* (1996) Birth weight for gestational age as a health indicator: birth weight and mortality measures at the local area level. *Eur. J. Public Health.* **6**:137–41.

84 Koupilova I, Vagero D, Leon DA *et al.* (1998) Social variation in size at birth and preterm delivery in the Czech Republic and Sweden, 1989–91. *Paediatr. Perinat. Epidemiol.* **12**:7–24.

85 Carr-Hill R (1988) Time trends in inequalities in health. *J. Biosoc. Sci.* **20**:253–63.

86 Tanner JM (1989) *Fetus into Man* (2e). Castlemead Publications, Ware, Herts.

87 Cernerud L (1991) *Growth and social conditions: height and weight of Stockholm children in a public health context.* NHV-Report 1991:5, The Nordic School of Public Health, Goteborg.

88 Miller FJW, Court SDM, Knox EG *et al.* (1974) *The School Years in Newcastle upon Tyne.* Oxford University Press, Oxford.

89 Lasker GW and Mascie-Taylor CGN (1989) Effects of social class differences and social mobility on growth and body mass index in a British cohort. *Ann. Hum. Biol.* **16**:1–8.

90 Voss LD, Mulligan J and Betts PR (1998) Short stature at school entry – an index of social deprivation? (The Wessex Growth Study) *Child: care, health and development.* **24**: 145–56.

91 Bielicki T (1986) Physical growth as a measure of the economic well-being of populations: the twentieth century. In *Human Growth* (2e) (eds F Falkner and JH Tanner). Plenum, New York.

92 Peck AMN and Vagero DH (1987) Adult body height and childhood socioeconomic group in the Swedish population. *J. Epidemiol. Community Health.* **41**:333–7.

93   Notkola V, Punsar S, Karvenon MJ *et al.* (1985) Socio-economic conditions in childhood and mortality and morbidity caused by coronary heart disease in adulthood in rural Finland. *Soc. Sci. Med.* **21**:517–23.

94   Waaler HTH (1984) Height, weight and mortality: the Norwegian experience. *Acta Med. Scand.* **Suppl. 679.**

95   Haggarty R, Roghmann K and Pless IB (1975) *Child Health in the Community.* Wiley, Chichester.

96   Rutter M and Smith D (eds) (1995) *Psychosocial Disorders in Young People.* Wiley, Chichester.

97   Lindstrom B and Kohler L (1995) Children and families in distress. In *Social Paediatrics* (eds B Lindstrom and NJ Spencer). Oxford University Press, Oxford.

98   Taylor J, Spencer NJ and Baldwin N (2000) The social, economic and political context of parenting. *Arch. Dis. Child.* **82**:113–20.

99   Murray C, Field F, Brown JC *et al.* (1990) *The Emerging British Underclass.* Institute of Economic Affairs Health and Welfare Unit, London.

100   Smith T (1993) Influence of socioeconomic factors on attaining targets for reducing teenage pregnancies. *BMJ.* **306**:1232–5.

101   Spencer NJ (1993) Teenage mothers. *Curr. Paediatr.* **4**: 48–51.

102   Brooks-Gunn J and Duncan GJ (1997) The effects of poverty on children. *The Future of Children.* **7**:55–71.

103   Wedge P and Prosser H (1973) *Born to Fail?* Arrow Books, London.

104   Mooney T (1998) Highs and lows of achievement. *Guardian Education*, Tuesday, December 1, p. 3.

105   Ross DP and Roberts P (1999) *Income and Child Well-being: A New Perspective on the Poverty Debate.* Canadian Council on Social Development, Ottawa, Canada.

106   Gray J and Jesson D (1990) *Truancy in Secondary Schools Amongst Fifth-year Pupils.* Educational Research Centre, Sheffield University, Sheffield.

107   Wolfe B (1990) *Is there economic discrimination against children?* Discussion Paper 904-900. Institute for Research on Poverty, Madison.

108   Bebbington A and Miles J (1989) The background of children who enter local authority care. *Br. J. Soc. Work.* **19**:349–68.

109   Hoghughi M and Speight ANP (1998) Good enough parenting for all children – a strategy for a healthier society. *Arch. Dis. Child.* **78**:293–6.

110   Baldwin N and Spencer NJ (1993) Deprivation and child abuse: implications for strategic planning in children's services. *Children and Society.* **7**:357–75.

111   Frost N (1990) Official intervention and child protection: the relationship between state and family in contemporary Britain. In *The Violence Against Children Study Group: Taking Child Abuse Seriously.* Unwin Hyman, London.

112   Hallet C (1993) Child abuse inquiries and public policy. In *Child Abuse: Public Policy and Professional Practice* (ed. O Stevenson). Harvester Wheatsheaf, Hemel Hempstead.

113   Sedlak A (1993) *Risk factors for child abuse and neglect in the US.* Paper presented at the Fourth European Conference on Child Abuse and Neglect, March 1993, Padua, Italy.

114   Frank DA and Zeisel SH (1988) Failure to thrive. *Pediatr. Clin. North Am.* **35**:1187–205.

115   Garrow J (1991) *Obesity and Overweight.* Health Education Authority, HMSO, London.

116 Parsons TJ, Power C, Logan S *et al.* (1999) Childhood predictors of adult obesity: a systematic review. *Int. J. Obesity.* **23**Suppl(8):S1–S107.

117 Bone M and Meltzer H (1989) *The prevalence of disability among children.* OPCS survey of disability in Great Britain: report 3. HMSO, London.

118 Department of Health (1998) *The Health of Young People 1995–97.* The Stationery Office, London.

119 Wadsworth MEJ (1991) *The Imprint of Time.* Clarendon Press, Oxford.

120 Scahill L, Schwab-Stone M, Merikangas KR *et al.* (1999) Psychosocial and clinical correlates of ADHD in a community sample of school-age children. *J. Am. Acad. Child Adolesc. Psychiat.* **38**:976–84.

121 Costello EJ, Angold A, Burns BJ *et al.* (1996) The Great Smoky Mountains Study of Youth. Goals, design, methods and the prevalence of DSM-III-R disorders. *Arch. Gen. Psychiat.* **53**:1129–36.

122 Parker S, Greer S and Zuckerman B (1988) Double jeopardy: the impact of poverty on early child development. *Pediatr. Clin. North Am.* **35**:1–14.

123 Brown GW and Harris T (1978) *Social Origins of Depression: A Study of Psychiatric Disorder in Women.* Tavistock, London.

124 Oakley A, Rigby AS and Hickey D (1993) Women and children last? Class, health and the role of maternal and child health services. *Eur. J. Public Health.* **3**:220–6.

125 Arber S (1987) Social class, non-employment and chronic illness: continuing the inequalities in health debate. *BMJ.* **294**:1069–74.

126 Townsend P and Davidson N (1982) *Inequalities in Health: The Black Report.* Penguin, Harmondsworth.

127 Pamuk ER (1988) Social class inequality in infant mortality in England and Wales from 1921 to 1980. *Eur. J. Popul.* **4**:1–21.

128 Phillimore P, Beattie A and Townsend P (1994) Widening health inequalities in northern England. *BMJ.* **308**:1125–8.

129 Roberts I and Power C (1996) Does the decline in child injury mortality vary by social class? A comparison of class-specific mortality in 1981 and 1991. *BMJ.* **313**:784–6.

130 Children's Defense Fund (1989) *A Children's Defense Budget.* Children's Defense Fund, Washington, DC.

131 Ciment J (1999) Health situation in the former Communist bloc dire, says Unicef. *BMJ.* **319**:1324.

132 Marmot MG and Smith GD (1989) Why are the Japanese living longer? *BMJ.* **299**:1547–51.

Part Three

The causal debate

7

'Race', ethnicity, poverty and child health

Introduction

'Race' and ethnicity are commonly used variables in health research. However, both are associated with problems of definition and confusion of sociocultural and biological concepts. These problems and confusions assume particular importance when the independent effects of 'race' and ethnicity on health are studied. As 'race' is so important in the debate on causal relations between poverty and child health in a number of countries in addition to the USA (for example Australia), the chapter is included in the causal mechanisms and debate section of the book. Following the convention used by Miles[1] and Ahmed,[2] 'race' appears in quotes as its scientific validity is questionable (*see* below).

The chapter examines the definitions and concepts underpinning 'race' and ethnicity with particular reference to their use in the study of the determinants of child health. Examples from the literature are used to illustrate the potential for inappropriate attribution of independent effects of 'race' and ethnicity on child health. Some general principles for the use of these variables in child health research are considered.

Definitions and concepts of 'race' and ethnicity

'Race' as a biological concept

Blumenbach, a professor of natural history at the University of Gottingen in Germany at the end of the 18th century, was the first to publish a systematic racial hierarchy and the first to publicise the term 'Caucasian'.[3] Following the naturalist, Buffon, who wrote earlier in the same century, Blumenbach conceived of the 'Caucasians' as the first and most talented 'race' from which all others had degenerated to become Chinese, Negroes etc.[3]

The origin of the term 'Caucasian' to describe white-skinned peoples is unclear. According to Bernal,[3] Blumenbach believed the Georgians to be the finest 'white race'. There were also religious reasons in that it was thought that Noah's Ark had landed on Mount Ararat in the Southern Caucasus as well as a German Romantic tendency to place the origins of mankind in the Eastern mountains of Europe, not in the river valleys of the Nile and the Euphrates as the ancients had believed. Subsequently, partial support has been lent to the 'Caucasian' concept by linguists who identify the Caucasus as the geographical origin of the so-called Proto–Indo–European (PIE) language.[4] However, as its name suggests, PIE is thought to be the origin of Indian subcontinental languages, thus including peoples who are now classified as 'Asian' or 'Black' in some classifications of 'race'/ethnicity.

By the mid-19th century, the dominant theory of 'race' had become established in scientific writings and asserted that the world's population is constituted by a number of different 'races'[1] though anthropologists continued to argue over the precise number.[5] Most classifications identified four 'races': Australoid, Mongoloid, Negroid and Caucasian. Anthropology textbooks earlier in the 20th century contained 'family trees' of the human development (*see* Figure 7.1) in which other 'races' were shown branching off early from a main stem of 'the basic white race' (Hooton 1947, quoted in [5]).

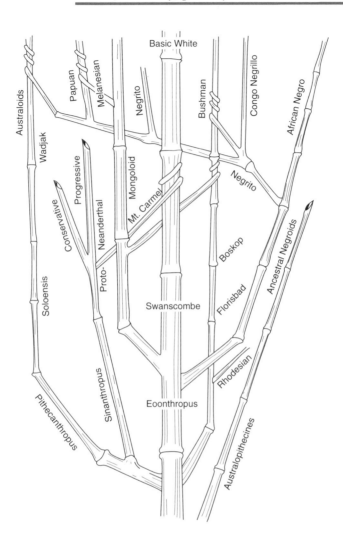

Figure 7.1 Family tree of man. (Source [5])

Concepts of 'race' came into their own with the establishment of nation states and the colonisation of other countries.[1] Sir Francis Younghusband, the leader of the British invasion of Tibet in 1904, demonstrates how useful the 'scientific' concept of 'race' was in justifying the subjugation of other peoples:

> *No European can mix with non-Christian races without feeling his moral superiority over them. He feels,*

from the first contact with them, that whatever may be their relative positions from an intellectual point of view, he is stronger morally than they are. And facts show that this feeling is a true one. It is not because we are any cleverer than the natives of India, because we have more brains or bigger heads than they have, that we rule India; but because we are stronger morally than they are. Our superiority over them is not due to mere sharpness of intellect, but to the higher moral nature to which we have attained in the development of the human race. (Younghusband, quoted in [6])

The racist 'science' which Younghusband uses to explain the right of Europeans to rule over peoples had always sought to equate social, moral and cultural features with biology. Josiah Nott, a physician in the southern states of America around the time of the civil war, wrote:

The Negro races stand at the lowest point in the scale of human beings ... It is clear they are incapable of self-government and that any attempt to improve their condition is warring against an immutable force of nature. (Nott, quoted in [7])

As with Younghusband, Nott seeks to justify slavery and its consequences on the basis that it is a 'natural' condition for peoples who are biologically incapable of self-government.

Long before the watershed of the use of pseudo-scientific racial theories by Nazism, the classifications and assumptions of racist 'science', particularly their use to support the concept of a biologically determined capacity for cultural development, had been challenged. Krieger[7] documents the opposition in medical circles to the concepts advanced by Nott, most notably from an emerging group of black physicians in America after 1860. Since 1945, the biological determination of cultural development has been scientifically discredited though 'scientific publications' based on these concepts continue to appear, claiming amongst other things an inherited basis for the differential educational achievements of different 'races' in the USA[8] and attributing the high levels of AIDS in Africa to the 'low marital stability and the permissive sexual attitudes of the Negroid race'.[9]

It is clear from the history of the classification of 'race' and its use in scientific literature that 'race' is primarily a social rather than a biological construct, serving the interests of dominant groups, particularly during the era of colonialism.[1,2,7] In biological terms, it describes a limited number of phenotypical differences, most notably skin colour; in fact what is being described is the distribution of gene frequencies across populations. Even these gene variations are greater within local populations (84% of genetic variation) than between the classically described 'races' (10% of genetic variation).[10,11] Thus, the commonly used racial categories are more alike than different in biological and genetic terms and cannot be unambiguously distinguished on any scientific criteria.

The variation in gene frequency between populations as well as the extent of common genes is understandable given that human history is one of migration.[4] Even before the 'shrinking' of the world in the second part of the 20th century associated with greatly facilitated world travel, migrations had been the norm rather than the exception, and concepts of 'racial purity' or even a common 'racial identity' become meaningless when examined against these patterns of migration. An inevitable consequence of migration is the mixing and change of gene pools and a consequent change in the patterns of gene variation in both the migrant and host populations.

Ethnicity

As part of the move away from racial classifications, the concept of ethnicity has been developed to examine the differences in health experience of different groups, particularly minority migrant groups within dominant cultures. In contrast to the original concepts of 'race', ethnicity is 'a social category referring to a shared heritage which includes a common geographical origin and history, distinctive language and a characteristic culture'.[12]

However, problems of definition have plagued these classifications. Firstly, ethnicity is often inappropriately used as a synonym for 'race'.[13] Secondly, ethnic classifications are often aggregate terms covering many cultures; for example, the term 'Asian', used in many UK studies, includes people from cultures as different as Pakistan and Sri Lanka, speaking a multitude of languages and practising a wide variety of religions. As McKenzie and Crowcroft[14] point out, 'most systems of classification would class all the warring factions in Bosnia as one ethnic group together with groups as culturally diverse as the Swedish and the Iranians (White/Caucasian) and ignore the diversity of cultural and religious life in Africa (Black African)'. Thirdly, culture changes rapidly and cannot be taken as a permanent and unchanging feature of a population, especially one that has migrated to another country where another culture is dominant. Cultures are in a dynamic relationship; migrants rapidly incorporate elements of the dominant culture and the dominant culture is influenced by elements of the migrant culture (for example, food culture in the UK has been greatly influenced by migrants from Italy, the Indian subcontinent [ISC] and China). This is well illustrated by the difficulties experienced in OPCS classifications related to mixed categories which were eventually dropped from the 1991 UK Census categories.[15] Fourthly, as with 'race', interpretation of results classified by ethnicity is influenced by ethnocentricity[13] which is the tendency to view one's own culture as the standard against which others are judged.

The confusion of biological and social categories

Though biological determinism based on 'race' has been generally discredited, the classification of 'race' continues to be extensively used in medical and social science research, generating annually 2500 papers on Medline,[14] and many of these papers continue to utilise categories such as 'Caucasoid', 'Negroid' and 'Mongoloid'.

Classifications of 'race'/ethnicity in current scientific literature vary with the country to which the classification is applied: in the UK, 'Caucasian' or 'white', 'Asian' (referring to those from the ISC) and 'Afro-Caribbean' are used amongst others; in the USA, 'white', 'black', 'Hispanic' and 'Native American' are the main categories in use.

Official classifications have changed in a way that reflects both the changes in populations but also the change in the political approach to 'race' and ethnicity. Skellington and Morris[16] list various classifications used in the UK: from 1970–82, the Department of Employment used the categories of East African, other African, West Indian, Indian, Pakistani, Bangladeshi and other Commonwealth countries to monitor what it called 'coloured' unemployment; the Labour Force Survey and the General Household Survey use white, West Indian or Guyanese, Indian, Pakistani, Bangladeshi, Chinese, African, Arabian, mixed or other; since 1975, the Metropolitan Police have used six classes: IC1 – white-skinned European types, IC2 – dark-skinned European types, IC3 – Negroid types, IC4 – Indians and Pakistanis, IC5 – Chinese and Mongolians, IC6 – Arabians; the 1991 Census asked people to select one of nine categories – white, black-Caribbean, black-African, black-other, Indian, Pakistani, Bangladeshi, Chinese or other.

The US Census Bureau has routinely changed its racial categories with no classification having been used in more than two censuses.[17] Up to the mid-1970s, most health data used the classification 'White' and 'non-White'. Subsequently the categories were expanded to include blacks, American Indians, Asian and Pacific Islanders and Hispanics.

The confusion inherent in many classifications is well illustrated by the following quote from a review of epidemiological research into the sudden infant death syndrome (SIDS):

Differences in SIDS rates have been observed between ethnic groups. Some of the rate difference between ethnic groups can be explained by differences in socio-economic status, and in fact the NICHD study showed that the higher SIDS rates for black Americans were entirely explained by this factor. However, the ethnic differences between Caucasians (3.9/1000 live births) and the more socially disadvantaged Pacific Islanders (1.9/1000) and Maoris (6.5/1000) in New Zealand cannot be explained in this way. In Birmingham, UK, the significantly lower risk of SIDS amongst Asians persisted after controlling for

> *maternal age, social class and birth weight. In California, the incidence of SIDS in Hispanics varied according to whether the mother was born in the USA (1.5/1000) or Mexico (0.8/1000). These findings suggest that culturally-related infant care practices may be an important determinant of SIDS.*[18]

Within this quotation it is evident that the classifications of 'race' and ethnicity are a confused jumble of biological and social categories, some of which remain rooted in the 'mind-set' of the discredited biological determinist classifications of 'race'. 'Black' refers to skin colour and is clearly a biological characteristic; 'Caucasian' is a term arising from the original classifications of racist science and presumably in this context refers to those of European origin; 'Asian' refers to people of ISC origin and is a lumping together of many different cultures; 'Hispanic' refers to those from Mexico and other Central American countries and islands such as Puerto Rico and is similarly a lumping together of many different cultures.

'Race' and ethnic differences in child health

Differences in child health outcomes by 'race' and ethnic group are well documented. In many cases, particularly amongst black groups and those from the ISC, ethnic minority children in most developed countries suffer more adverse child health outcomes than those of the dominant ethnic group: in the UK, births to mothers born in Pakistan show persistently higher rates of perinatal mortality and lower birth weights;[19] in the USA, black American children have increased adverse outcomes[20] across a range of child health problems from birth weight (twice the low birth weight rate of white Americans) to asthma and persistent wheeze;[21] Maoris in New Zealand[22,23] and Aboriginals in Australia[24,25] show similar increased levels of adverse outcomes, particularly in infancy and early childhood. The evidence for 'racial'/ethnic minority group differences in child health is fully reviewed elsewhere.[19,20,24,26] In this chapter, the main focus is the explanations for these differences.

Biological explanations

Biological explanations are most tenable in relation to the diseases related directly to variation in genetic pools. As discussed above, ethnic groups tend to hold certain genes in common. Although these commonly held genes explain only approximately 10% of gene variation, they are responsible for some characteristic phenotypical features such as skin colour and they predispose individuals within these populations to particular inherited diseases. Many of these diseases are recessively inherited with the carrier state conferring some advantage; the best known example is sickling trait, the carrier state of sickle cell disease, which is thought to protect against malaria. Ethnocentricity tends to lead those in Western societies to think of these conditions as 'exotic' and only affecting other ethnic groups.[27] All peoples holding common gene pools are subject to particular diseases: in those of northern European origin, cystic fibrosis is one of the best known.

Despite their importance as individual conditions, these diseases contribute little to the overall differences in health between 'races' and ethnic groups. For example, it has been estimated that sickle cell anaemia accounts for only 0.3% of the total number of excess deaths in the black American population.[28]

The so-called 'tropical' diseases tend to be seen as associated with particular ethnic groups and have become part of the perception of a biological susceptibility to specific diseases. Apart from those diseases which are linked with very specific environmental conditions and depend for their perpetuation on those conditions, the majority of diseases afflicting people in tropical areas are diseases of poverty and were prevalent in developed countries in the 19th century (*see* Chapters 4 and 5). Some of these diseases, such as TB, are still present in developed countries and continue to be associated with poverty and overcrowded living conditions.[29,30] As socio-economic conditions improve in some regions of 'tropical' countries,[31] the prevalence of these diseases falls.[32]

'Genetic racial differences' have been advanced to explain birth weight differences between infants of European and Aboriginal origin in Australia[25] and between black and white

Americans.[20] Differences in the genetic pool are thought to account for the difference in height noted between children in Hong Kong and children of European and African–American origin.[33] Social and environmental factors interact with genetic factors. However, as Figure 5.8 (see p. 119) shows, these social influences are stronger in most countries, with the exception of Hong Kong, with boys of high income groups achieving heights equivalent to the median for the US population.[34]

Japanese children growing up in San Francisco in the 1950s were noted to be taller than those growing up in Japan;[35] however, there is now no difference in height between Japanese growing up in Japan and California but they remain at about the 15th centile of the British standards[33] suggesting that improvements in socio-economic circumstances have increased height in this group though they remain smaller as a consequence of the effects of their genetic pool. By contrast, Sikh boys and girls in Walsall were 3 cm and 1.5 cm taller at the age of five years than European boys and girls,[36] indicating that this economically successful group were not impeded by genetic factors in growth compared with other groups.

Further evidence of the weakness of genetic influences on some child health outcomes arises from studies of maternal nativity status which demonstrate marked differences in mortality rates between infants of US-born Puerto Rican mothers and those born in Puerto Rico[37] and infants of US-born black mothers and foreign-born black mothers.[38] Though presumably from the same genetic pool, the socio-economic and cultural differences between the groups lead to different outcomes for their infants.

Cultural explanations

Cultural factors play a part in disease susceptibility.[12] However, as Smaje points out:

> *Culture is typically invoked in a residual and undifferentiated way as an independent variable, with little effort expended in postulating which particular aspects of culture may be injurious or protective to health.*
> ([26] p. 85)

Consanguinity is one of the cultural factors which is often invoked[39] to explain differences between infants of Pakistani origin and other ethnic groups in the incidence of congenital abnormalities which account for about half of the excess of perinatal and post-neonatal deaths in these infants.[19] However, when specific conditions such as fetal growth,[40] cardiac abnormalities[41] and hypothyroidism[42] are examined, the contribution of consanguinity to the observed differences is small. Honeyman *et al.*[40] review the literature on the effects of parental consanguinity on fetal growth and demonstrate that only two out of seven studies showed significant differences related to consanguinity. A study conducted in Lahore, Pakistan[43] showed that consanguinity and low socio-economic status were closely correlated and both were associated with increased risk of birth defects. When socio-economic status was accounted for there was no residual effect of consanguinity. This may be an effect of socio-economic status of family of origin. It is clear that, despite the commonly held view to the contrary, the principal importance of consanguinity in the explanation of observed differences has yet to be established.[19]

Diet has been suggested as a 'cultural' explanation for ethnic health differences. For example, nutritional rickets is more prevalent in the UK among the children of families from the ISC than in children of European origin.[44,45] This difference has been attributed to 'Asian' diets low in vitamin D and the condition has come to be known as 'Asian rickets'.[46] This attribution and the associated misnomer fail to take account of the prevalence of rickets amongst children in European countries in the 19th century and the vitamin D supplementation of margarine which is largely responsible for the elimination of the disease in the 'indigenous' population since the Second World War. Many families from the ISC cook with ghee and margarine is not widely used. A proposal to fortify chappati flour with vitamin D was rejected.[47]

A debate has developed around the observation, first made in studies in New Zealand, that bed sharing may be a risk factor for SIDS.[23] Bed sharing is more prevalent amongst Maori families than those of northern European origin and is only a risk factor in this ethnic group.[23] When confounding factors are accounted for, the effect of bed sharing disappears.[48] Bed sharing occurs in 90% of the world's population[48] but in Western industrialised societies it has come to be considered as undesirable and infants are expected to develop an adult pattern of sleep by three to four months of age. Continuous close proximity of the infant with the adults in the household may be protective and may be part of the explanation for the very low SIDS rate noted among infants of Bangladeshi mothers in the UK.[49]

The assumptions related to consanguinity, diet and bed sharing illustrate an ethnocentric tendency in the interpretation of research findings. On available evidence, cultural factors explain little of the major differences in child health between ethnic groups. Differences within ethnic groups are greater than those between groups, with the economically advantaged in each ethnic group showing a health advantage over less privileged members of the same group.

Socio-economic explanations

In most 'Western' countries, black and ethnic minority people are overtly and covertly discriminated against in many aspects of social and economic life, resulting in limited opportunities and lower socio-economic status (SES).[12,19,50,51] Ethnic minority status itself does not automatically imply disadvantage; the white South African population are an ethnic minority but their economic and social dominance, maintained by force, has ensured that it is the black majority whose opportunities have been limited and whose socio-economic position has been low. Neither is the problem of discrimination confined to migrants; the white South African population are migrants as are the white populations of New Zealand, Australia and the USA. In these situations the migrant populations, having conquered and colonised (and in some cases slaughtered) the indigenous peoples, have discriminated against them and ensured their continuing social and economic disadvantage. As Susser *et al.* point out:

> *In societies influenced by legacies of slavery or colonialism or both, racial and ethnic divisions tend*

to coincide with those of the class structure ... Where racial disadvantage is present, however, it can be largely explained by the close association of minority status – in the United States, being black especially – with lower class membership. For such groups, the two types of status are conflated and, technically, confounded. Race may operate over and above class, however, usually exaggerating and occasionally suppressing differences between groups. ([12] p. 245)

In the USA, the links between low SES and 'race' are well documented.[17,51,52] Using the Human Development Index (HDI) developed by the United Nations Development Project,[31] white Americans have a HDI of 0.986 compared with 0.881 for black Americans. The GDP per capita, expressed as purchasing power parity dollars (PPP$), for black Americans was 17 100 in 1993 compared with 22 000 for white Americans.[31] In 1990, 21.9% of US children were living on or below the official poverty line; however, for black American and hispanic American children the rates are much higher – 43.5% and 37.6% respectively.[52] Between three to five million of US children live in persistent poverty with family incomes on average US$4500 below the poverty line, and the majority of these children are black. 'Race' has been a substitute for social class, and to some extent poverty, in official US statistics.[51,53]

In the UK, similar links have been noted between ethnicity and low SES. Unemployment rates for most minority ethnic groups, with the exception of the Chinese and East African Indians, are higher than those of European origin and have increased through the period of recession in the 1980s;[26] low-paid occupations employ a disproportionately high number of people from ethnic minority groups and, on average, male earnings of Indians and East African Indians are less than those of European origin with Caribbeans earning less still and Pakistanis and Bangladeshis earning the least;[50] ethnic minority workers are more likely to experience poor working conditions;[26] a higher proportion of people of Indian and Pakistani origin are home owner-occupiers than those of European origin but peoples of Caribbean and Bangladeshi origin are more likely to rent from local authorities, and the quality of housing in each category of tenure tends to be poorer.[26]

South Africa is an untypical case because of the policy of apartheid practised by the National Party government until the recent elections. However, the close links between 'race' and socio-economic status in South Africa serve to illustrate the role of institutionalised racism in creating disadvantaged groups almost entirely on the basis of skin colour and the complexities of disentangling 'race' from poverty. The HDI for black South Africans is 0.462 (on a par with the Congo) compared with 0.878 (on a par with Spain) for white South Africans. Poverty is one of the main determinants of this difference: GDP per capita for black South Africans is 1710 PPP$ as against 14 920 PPP$ for their white fellow citizens (*see* Chapter 5).

As a direct result of colonialism and the slave trade, ethnic minority groups, distinguishable by their skin colour or distinctive culture, have tended to occupy low social positions and been subjected to long-standing discrimination which serves to maintain their disadvantaged status. Within each social group, those from ethnic minorities tend to be the most disadvantaged though there are some clear exceptions to this general rule, such as the Japanese Americans[12] and the Sikhs in the UK.[36]

This long-standing link of ethnic minority populations with poverty (in their native countries as well as the host country) and disadvantage inevitably leads to confounding of 'race' and ethnicity and SES in socio-medical and epidemiological research.[12,19,51,54] Studies which have attempted to account for SES have shown a reduction in the health differential between ethnic groups;[19,55,56] however, residual differences continue to be noted after adjustment for SES.[17,22,57]

Making sense of these explanations

It is evident from the above that socio-economic factors are amongst the most powerful determinants of the health differentials noted between 'races' and ethnic groups. However, there are unexplained differences after adjustment. Biological factors may account for some of these unexplained differences but only in relation to the small number of conditions which are mediated by differences in gene frequency between populations. Cultural factors have been shown to influence some health outcomes, sometimes to the advantage of minority ethnic groups; however, culture varies as much within ethnic groups as between them with large differences in practices depending on geography and social status, making it unlikely that often unspecified cultural factors account for these residual differences.

More plausible reasons for the persistence of apparent 'race' and ethnic differences after accounting for SES are likely to lie in the methodological inadequacies of the studies themselves and specifically the classification of 'race', ethnic and SES variables.

The potential for residual confounding is high when variables are ill- or poorly defined.[58] Given that both SES and 'race'/ethnicity variables are frequently ill-defined, often by the 'lumping' of categories which conceals major intra-group differences, residual confounding is likely to account for some of the unexplained residuum of 'race' and ethnic health differences.

The Registrar General's Social Class (RGSC), the classification most commonly used in the UK and in other countries such as Australia and New Zealand, is a very crude measure of SES[59] and is particularly unsuitable for use in studying the interaction with ethnicity as those in ethnic minority groups are likely to be in the lower grades of all occupations.[50] Ethnicity will pick out the most deprived in each social class and will appear to have a residual effect which may be due in reality to the overall lower within-class position of ethnic minority groups. US studies which have used the poverty line as the measure of SES are likely to suffer the same problems of adjusting; families move in and out of poverty and black American children are much more likely to live in families in chronic and severe poverty with incomes well below the federal poverty line.[52]

Current SES is frequently treated in studies as the sole and key socio-economic health determinant; however, health is determined by experience over the life course and differences in early life experience of children and the life experience of their parents are likely to bear on child health outcomes. The accumulated experiences of low SES are likely to affect ethnic minority groups more than dominant groups. This is especially likely to be true in countries, such as the USA and the UK, in which slavery and colonial domination have played such an important role in the political and social relations between minority and dominant groups.

Very few studies have attempted to quantify the combined effects of poverty and discrimination – 'double jeopardy' – on ethnic minority children and families; available evidence suggests that racial discrimination and the internalisation of racist ideology by minority group members are adversely linked to physical and mental health.[60,61] Discrimination in employment and health service delivery in the UK NHS is well documented[62,63] and others[2,27] have shown how racism influences research questions and conclusions. In discussing the interaction of 'race' and health, a number of authors have considered the possible role of discrimination in explaining residual adverse risk of 'race' following adjustment for SES. Pearson states:

> *Social class is a very crude measure of socio-economic position and resources, and may be particularly inadequate as such a measure for minorities, as they are more likely to be in the lower grades of all occupations and to experience discrimination in other relevant areas of social and material life.* ([19] p. 89)

Using 'race' and ethnicity variables in socio-medical research

It is tempting in view of the obvious flaws both in biological and social classifications to abandon them entirely on the grounds that those based on biological differences are racist and those based on culture fail to reflect real cultural diversity and are prone to ethnocentricity[1,15] and much of the variation in health outcomes is anyway explained by long-standing socio-economic disadvantage and discrimination. Whilst there is no doubt that classifications of 'race' were underpinned by racist and colonialist concepts[3] and were used to justify maltreatment of colonised peoples, there is a strong case for categories which allow a distinction to be made between the health and other experiences of host and migrant populations in order to monitor the effects of racism on health[17] and provide data to inform service provision related to conditions, such as sickle cell disease, to which some populations are more vulnerable as a result of shared gene pools.

If ethnic classifications are to be used in research or in the collection of routine population data, the users should have clear aims in the use of the categories and follow the 'good practice' guidelines laid down by Senior and Bhopal.[13] They call for the improvement of the value of ethnicity as an epidemiological variable by wider recognition of its limitations, acknowledgement and avoidance of ethnocentricity, consideration of the confounding effects of socio-economic factors, prioritisation of research into ethnic classification and recognition of the fluidity and dynamic nature of culture and ethnicity.

There is an urgent need to develop SES measures which are sensitive to the potential cumulative effects of discrimination and long-standing disadvantage.[17,19] The extent to which various SES measures may be differently predictive of health outcome for different populations, and the interaction of SES with migration experience and acculturative stress, need to be addressed.[17] Skin colour itself has been shown to be a powerful marker of SES;[17] income, education and occupational status were found to be inversely related to darker skin colour in a national representative sample of African–Americans, and skin colour was a stronger predictor of adult occupational status and income than parental SES.[64] This finding correlates with the role of discrimination and racism in the continued low relative socio-economic position of ethnic minority groups with dark skin.

Summary

1   'Race' is a socially constructed rather than a biological concept.

2   Biological determinism in relation to health has been largely discredited.

3   Classifications of 'race' and ethnicity in socio-medical literature frequently represent a confusion between biological and socio-cultural concepts, and researchers have a duty to explicitly define their terms.

4   In many Western countries, ethnic minority groups, particularly those distinguished by dark skin colour, have a lower socio-economic status and poverty is more common amongst them than amongst the 'host' population. Within each socio-economic group, ethnic minority peoples tend to occupy the lower end so that there is a disproportionate number of children of ethnic minority groups living in severe or chronic socio-economic disadvantage.

5   Children of ethnic minority groups suffer more adverse health outcomes. However, their adverse socio-economic circumstances seem to explain more of this differential than biological or cultural factors. Those who are economically advantaged from minority cultures and ethnic groups have health outcomes similar to those of the economically advantaged in the dominant cultural group.

6   Commonly used measures of SES, such as occupational group, are inadequate for studying the complex relationship between ethnicity, socio-economic factors and health. Measures sensitive to the effects of discrimination and long-standing disadvantage need to be developed. Caution must be exercised in the interpretation of results derived from studies adjusting for SES using traditional measures; the potential for residual confounding is particularly high given the lack of precision of both the 'race'/ethnicity and the SES variables.

References

1   Miles R (1993) *Racism After 'Race Relations'*. Routledge, London.

2   Ahmed W (1993) *'Race' and Health in Contemporary Britain*. Open University Press, Milton Keynes.

3   Bernal M (1987) *Black Athena: The Afroasiatic Roots of Classical Civilisation*. Vintage, London.

4   Diamond J (1991) *The Rise and Fall of the Third Chimpanzee*. Vintage, London.

5   Leslie C (1990) Scientific racism: reflections on peer review, science and ideology. *Soc. Sci. Med.* **31**:891–912.

6   Huttenback RA (1976) *Racism and Empire: White Settlers and Colored Immigrants in British Self-governing Colonies, 1830–1910*. Cornell University Press, Ithaca and London.

7   Kreiger N (1987) Theoretical underpinnings of the medical controversy on black/white differences in the United States. *Int. J. Health Serv.* **17**:259–78.

8   Murray C and Herrnstein R (1994) *The Bell Curve: Intelligence and Class Structure in American Life*. The Free Press, New York.

9   Rushton P and Bogaert AF (1989) Population differences in susceptibility to AIDS: an evolutionary analysis. *Soc. Sci. Med.* **28**:1211–20.

10 Jones JS (1981) How different are human races? *Nature.* **293**:188–90.

11 Lewontin R (1982) *Human Diversity.* Scientific American Books, New York.

12 Susser MW, Watson W and Hopper K (1985) *Sociology in Medicine* (3e). Oxford University Press, New York.

13 Senior PA and Bhopal R (1994) Ethnicity as a variable in epidemiological research. *BMJ.* **309**:327–30.

14 McKenzie KJ and Crowcroft NS (1994) Race, ethnicity, culture and science. *BMJ.* **309**:286–7.

15 Nanton P (1992) Official statistics and problems of inappropriate ethnic categorisation. *Policy and Politics.* **20**:277–85.

16 Skellington R and Morris P (1993) *'Race' in Britain Today.* Open University Press, Milton Keynes.

17 Williams D (1996) Race/ethnicity and socio-economic status: measurement and methodological issues. *Int. J. Health Serv.* **26**:483–505.

18 Dwyer T and Ponsonby A-L (1992) Sudden infant death syndrome – insights from epidemiological research. *J. Epidemiol. Community Health.* **46**:98–102.

19 Pearson M (1991) Ethnic differences in infant health. *Arch. Dis. Child.* **66**:88–90.

20 Starfield B and Budetti PP (1985) Child health status and risk factors. *Health Serv. Res.* **19**:817–86.

21 Schwartz J, Gold D, Dockery DW *et al.* (1990) Predictors of asthma and persistent wheeze in a national sample of children in the United States. *Am. Rev. Respir. Dis.* **142**:555–62.

22 Davis P (1984) Health patterns in New Zealand: class, ethnicity and the impact of economic development. *Soc. Sci. Med.* **18**:919–25.

23 Scragg R, Mitchell EA, Taylor BJ *et al.* (1993) Bed sharing, smoking and alcohol in the sudden infant death syndrome. *BMJ.* **307**:1312–18.

24 Jolly DL (1990) *The Impact of Adversity on Child Health – Poverty and Disadvantage.* Austalian College of Paediatrics, Parkville, Victoria.

25 Seward JF and Stanley FJ (1981) Comparison of births to Aboriginal and Caucasian mothers in Western Australia. *Med. J. Aust.* **2**:80–4.

26 Smaje C (1995) *Health, 'Race' and Ethnicity: Making Sense of the Evidence.* King's Fund Institute, London.

27 Donovan JL (1984) Ethnicity and health: a research review. *Soc. Sci. Med.* **19**:663–70.

28 Cooper R and David R (1986) The biological concept of race and its application to public health and epidemiology. *J. Health Politics, Policy and Law.* **11**:97–116.

29 Bhatti N, Law MR, Morris JK *et al.* (1995) Increasing incidence of tuberculosis in England and Wales: a study of the likely causes. *BMJ.* **310**:967–70.

30 Mangtani P, Jolley DJ, Watson JM *et al.* (1995) Socio-economic deprivation and notification rates for tuberculosis in London during 1982–91. *BMJ.* **310**:963–6.

31 United Nations Development Programme (1994) *Human Development Report 1994.* UNDP & Oxford University Press, New York.

32 Grant J (1994) *The State of the World's Children 1994.* Oxford University Press for Unicef, New York.

33 Tanner JM (1989) *Fetus into Man* (2e). Castlemead Publications, Ware, Herts.

34 Martorell R (1984) Genetics, environment and growth: issues in the assessment of nutritional status. In *Genetic Factors in Nutrition* (eds A Velasquez and H Bourges). Academic Press, New York.

35 Greulich WM (1976) Some secular changes in the growth of American-born and native Japanese children. *Am. J. Phys. Anthropol.* **45**:553–68.

36 Gatrad AR, Birch N and Hughes M (1994) Preschool weights and heights of Europeans and five subgroups of Asians in Britain. *Arch. Dis. Child.* **71**:207–10.

37 Engel T, Alexander GR and Leland NL (1995) Pregnancy outcomes of US-born Puerto Ricans: the role of maternal nativity status. *Am. J. Prev. Med.* **11**:34–9.

38 Kleinman JC, Fingerhut MA and Prager K (1991) Differences in infant mortality by race, nativity status and other maternal characteristics. *Am. J. Dis. Child.* **145**:194–9.

39　Terry PB, Bissenden JG, Condie RG *et al.* (1985) Ethnic differences in congenital malformations. *Arch. Dis. Child.* 60:866–8.

40　Honeyman MM, Bahl L, Marshall T *et al.* (1987) Consanguinity and fetal growth in Pakistani Moslems. *Arch. Dis. Child.* 62:1204–8.

41　Gatrad AR, Read AP and Watson GH (1984) Consanguinity and complex cardiac anomalies with situs ambiguus. *Arch. Dis. Child.* 59:242–5.

42　Rosenthal M, Addison GM and Price DA (1988) Congenital hypothyroidism: increased incidence in Asian families. *Arch. Dis. Child.* 63:790–3.

43　Yaqoob M, Gustavson KH, Jalil F *et al.* (1993) Early child health in Lahore, Pakistan. 2. Inbreeding. *Acta Paediatr. Scand.* 82(10):S17–26.

44　Goel K *et al.* (1976) Florid and sub-clinical rickets among immigrant children in Glasgow. *Lancet.* i:1141–3.

45　Ford JA, McIntosh WV, Butterfield R *et al.* (1976) Clinical and sub-clinical vitamin-D deficiency in Bradford children. *Arch. Dis. Child.* 51:939–43.

46　Goel K, Campbell S, Logan R *et al.* (1981) Reduced prevalence of rickets in Asian children in Glasgow. *Lancet.* ii:405–7.

47　Department of Health and Social Security (DHSS) (1980) *Rickets and osteomalacia. Report of the Working Party on Fortification of Foods with Vitamin D.* Committee on Medical Aspects of Food Policy. HMSO, London.

48　Klonoff-Cohen H and Edelstein SL (1995) Bed sharing and the sudden infant death syndrome. *BMJ.* 311:1269–72.

49　Gantley M, Davies DP and Murcott A (1993) Sudden infant death syndrome: links with infant care practices. *BMJ.* 306:16–20.

50 Brown C (1984) *Black and White Britain: The Third PSI Survey.* Heinemann, London.

51 Navarro V (1990) Race or class versus race and class: mortality differentials in the United States. *Lancet.* **336**:1238–40.

52 Danziger S and Stern J (1990) *The causes and consequences of child poverty in the United States.* Innocenti Occasional Papers, No. 10. Unicef International Child Development Centre, Florence, Italy.

53 Kreiger N and Fee E (1994) Social class: the missing link in US health data. *Int. J. Health Serv.* **24**:25–44.

54 Senior PA and Bhopal R (1994) Ethnicity as a variable in epidemiological research. *BMJ.* **309**:327–30.

55 Kraus JF, Peterson DR, Standfast SJ *et al.* (1988) The relationship of socioeconomic status and sudden infant death syndrome: confounding or effect modifier. In *Sudden Infant Death Syndrome: Risk Factors and Basic Mechanisms* (eds RM Harper and HJ Hoffman). PMA Publishing Corp., New York.

56 Rawlings JS and Weir MR (1992) Race- and rank-specific infant mortality in a US military polulation. *Am. J. Dis. Child.* **146**:313–16.

57 Kyle D, Sunderland R, Stonehouse M *et al.* (1990) Ethnic differences in incidence of sudden infant death syndrome. *Arch. Dis. Child.* **65**:830–3.

58 Smith GD and Phillips AN (1992) Confounding in epidemiological studies: why 'independent effects may not be all they seem. *BMJ.* **305**:757–9.

59 Smith GD, Blane D and Bartley M (1994) Explanations of socioeconomic differences in mortality: evidence from Britain and elsewhere. *Eur. J. Public Health.* **4**:131–44.

60 Kreiger N, Rowley DL, Herman AA *et al.* (1993) Racism, sexism and social class: implications for studies of health. *Am. J. Prev. Med.* **9**:82–122.

61 Williams D and Collins C (1995) US socioeconomic and racial differences in health: patterns and explanations. *Ann. Rev. Soc.* **21**:349–86.

62 Kushnik L (1988) Racism, the National Health Service and the health of black people. *Int. J. Health Serv.* **18**:457–70.

63 Esmail A and Etherington S (1993) Racial discrimination against doctors from ethnic minorities. *BMJ.* **306**:691–2.

64 Keith VM and Herring C (1991) Skin tone and stratification in the black community. *Am. J. Sociol.* **97**:760–78.

8

The causal debate

Introduction

As the chapters in the preceding section illustrate, there is overwhelming evidence to support the link between low socio-economic status (SES) and adverse health outcomes, particularly in childhood. Few socio-medical researchers would dispute this link. However, there is a major causal debate which has continued for many years. Four principal schools of thought have emerged: the artefact school; the social selection/mobility school; the behavioural/cultural school; the structural/materialist school. These schools of socio-medical thought are part of a wider political debate centring on the role of the individual in society and the responsibility of the state and government for the welfare of its more vulnerable citizens.

This chapter considers the various schools of thought in the causal debate before focusing on the two major schools – behavioural/cultural and structural/materialist. These schools and the causal debate are considered using three examples of particular importance to child health: parental smoking and early childhood illness; family diet, nutrition and child health; hygiene and child health in less developed countries and in developed countries in the 19th century. A particular focus is the contribution of the interpretation of the results of socio-medical research to the current emphasis on behavioural change among parents as the main way of improving child health, and key methodological issues which influence interpretation.

Explanations of health inequalities

Four conflicting explanations have been advanced to account for the social class gradient in adverse health outcomes: artefact; social selection; behavioural/cultural; structural/materialist.[1,2]

Artefact explanations

These suggest that the socio-economic gradient in health results from artefacts of measurement. Artefact explanations have been advanced in the UK and relate mainly to problems associated with the Registrar General's Social Class (RGSC) (*see* Chapter 1, p. 20). They include numerator–denominator bias, RGSC categorisation, changing size of social class groups, measures of socio-economic position, measures of ill health and measures of mortality.[2] Even within the UK context, none of these explanations can account for the consistent social class mortality differentials found in many studies.[2] Examined against the wealth of international and historical evidence considered in Chapters 4, 5 and 6, they are seen to have a narrow national focus and are totally inadequate to explain the consistent socio-economic differentials in mortality and morbidity noted in different countries using a variety of different measures of SES.

Social selection

Explanations based on social selection seek to explain socio-economic gradients in health on the basis that health determines social position rather than the reverse. Smith and co-workers identify two main explanations which fall within this category: intra-generational selection – sick individuals drifting down the social hierarchy and healthy individuals moving up; inter-generational selection – sick children tending to move to a social class position lower than that of their childhood.[2] Social selection has been shown, particularly in longitudinal studies, to explain little of the difference between socio-economic groups.[2-4]

Behavioural and cultural explanations

Behavioural and cultural explanations of socio-economic differentials in health have become dominant in recent years and are based on the premise that observed health differences between social groups are accounted for by health-related behaviour.[2,5] As a result, particularly in the developed world, socio-medical research has become focused on health-related behaviours, particularly smoking and diet.[2] In child health research, parental (particularly maternal) smoking and other health-related behaviours have been implicated in most major adverse health outcomes of pregnancy, infancy and early childhood, and the view that these behaviours account for observed SES differences now has wide currency.[6] Behavioural explanations have profoundly influenced health policy in some developed countries: health gain is expected to accrue mainly through behaviour change.[5,7]

Structural or life circumstances explanations

The Black Report and the more recent Acheson Report on health inequalities in the UK conclude that explanations based on the structure of society and inequalities of income distribution and opportunity best explain observed socio-economic differentials.[1,8] In other words, life circumstances, over which many people have little or no control, are responsible in a variety of ways and through a variety of mechanisms for health inequalities. In sharp contrast to the behavioural explanations, these imply a need for structural changes in society to reduce inequalities of income distribution and empower those disempowered by low SES and its consequent deprivations. As discussed in Chapter 5, poor countries which have adopted this general philosophy have been successful, despite their lack of economic wealth, in making remarkable improvements in the health status of their populations.[9]

The behavioural versus structural debate

The causal debate has centred on the structural and behavioural schools. For the reasons presented above, in my view and that of others, the artefact and social selection explanations are unable to account for more than a very small part of the observed health differentials and can be broadly dismissed. The behavioural versus structural debate in the context of child health is explored using three examples: parental smoking and child health; nutrition and choice in poor families; hygiene and cultural factors in less developed countries and in today's developed countries earlier in the 20th century. Hygiene and cultural factors in less developed countries have already been considered in Chapter 5 but are worth revisiting as they show how the causal debate is not confined to the developed world, where the effects of poverty are less obvious. Evidence from studies of adult health substantiate the conclusions drawn from the examples.

Parental smoking and child health

Smoking by parents, in particular mothers during pregnancy, has been implicated in many adverse pregnancy and early childhood health outcomes: early pregnancy miscarriage; low birth weight; respiratory disease in childhood; sudden infant death syndrome (SIDS); developmental delay.[10-15] Many of these outcomes are also linked with low SES (*see* Chapter 6).

Smoking itself is now very strongly linked to SES in most developed countries (*see* Table 8.1). A recent comprehensive literature review concludes:

> *Smoking prevalence can be demonstrated to vary with many different demographic and social characteristics. To a large extent it is collinear with social disadvantage at the individual level (for example young age, low educational attainments, high stress and depression), the immediate environment (housing circumstances and tenure, family structure, social*

Table 8.1   Trends in women's smoking and socio-economic status in Denmark (1970–87) and UK (1950–90). (Source [25] pp. 248–9)

	UK		Denmark	
	1950	*1990*	*1970*	*1987*
Higher social class/ occupational group	44%	14%	55%	39%
Lower social class/ occupational group	43%	36%	61%	58%

> *support) and in the wider perspective (access to amenities, social isolation and unemployment). There is evidence of a biological gradient in the relationship between smoking and disadvantage, with higher rates and level of smoking associated with more disadvantageous social and environmental circumstances.* ([16] p. 109)

The biological gradient mentioned in the above quote is illustrated by the linear gradient between amount smoked among mothers of small infants and levels of disadvantage shown in Figure 8.1.[17] Among mothers on income support, Graham and Blackburn[18] report the odds of being a smoker, adjusted for other socio-demographic variables, were 2.2 higher for mothers who had been on income support for more than five years compared with those who had been on income support less than a year.

Thus, SES is a powerful confounder of the relationship between smoking and child health. Adjustment for confounding by SES using conventional measures, such as occupational class of the head of the household, that do not take account of gradients within disadvantaged groups themselves, is likely to be susceptible to residual confounding.[18]

Adherents of the behavioural school have characterised parental smoking as 'the single most preventable cause of child illness', accounting for much or all of the SES differences in these outcomes.[6,12,14] These authors conclude that SES differences are

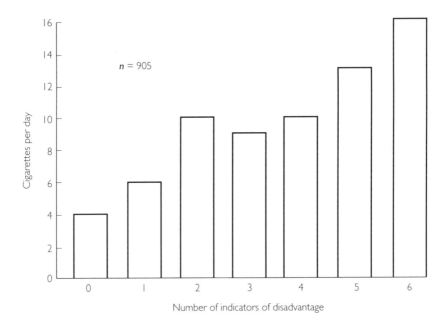

Figure 8.1   Relationship between deprivation and level of smoking. (Source [17])

accounted for by parental smoking because the association between parental smoking and the outcome of interest remains after standardisation for SES. Evidence for a causal relationship beyond mere statistical correlation has been advanced based on Bradford-Hill's criteria for establishing causal relationships.[19] Passive smoking by the fetus and the infant shows an apparent dose-related response for low birth weight (LBW) and SIDS.[12,20] Pathophysiological mechanisms have been advanced to support the biological plausibility of the relationship.[21]

These research conclusions and interpretations have been extremely influential and have been incorporated into health policy and health promotion programmes, such as the 'Back to Sleep Campaign' designed to reduce SIDS by promoting supine sleeping, non-smoking and avoidance of overwrapping.[22] With a few notable exceptions, health promotion materials and campaigns have chosen to ignore the social context in which both the adverse outcomes and the health-related behaviours occur.[23]

Despite the apparent strength of the correlation between parental smoking and adverse child health outcomes, there are a number of reasons for challenging the assertion that this correlation explains inequalities in child health outcomes such as LBW, SIDS and respiratory disease. In the UK, smoking among women is a relatively recent phenomenon, only becoming established after the Second World War, and the social class gradient was absent in 1958 and possibly reversed before then.[24] Though now showing some evidence of change, the social class gradient in women's smoking was until recently reversed in Spain and Greece; in both countries, the women in professional groups were more likely to smoke than their peers in lower social groups (*see* Table 8.2).[25-27]

Smoking among women in less developed countries is an even more recent phenomenon and in many countries it remains rare. As shown in the preceding section of this book (Chapters 4, 5 and 6), the links between SES and many adverse child health outcomes, including LBW, post-neonatal mortality and lower respiratory tract disease, long predated the advent of women's smoking on a large scale and have always been in the same direction whatever the direction of the social gradient of smoking. The same historical implausibility has been shown in relation to social class differentials in 'all-cause' adult male mortality in the UK, which have remained unchanged despite the change in the social class gradient in male smoking

Table 8.2 Smoking and socio-economic status in Spain, Greece and Italy. (Source [25])

	Italy (1986)	Spain (1987)	Greece (1980)
	%	%	%
Higher social/ educational group	30*	29.7	46
Middle social/ educational group	23*	22.7	48
Low social/ educational group	18*	11.2	41

* Age-adjusted prevalence.

since the 1950s.[2] The methodologies of many of the studies which conclude that passive smoking in pregnancy and childhood 'explains' SES differentials are flawed in various ways, leading to an overestimation of the effect of smoking on the outcomes under study. The commonest problem is *misclassification* of SES, increasing the potential for *residual confounding*, which occurs when one or more of the confounding variables in a study is inadequately classified, resulting in a systematic tendency to under- or overestimate its independent effect.[2,28,29] The shortcomings of social class categories, such as the RGSC used in the UK, based on occupation of the male head of the household, especially when studying maternal and child health outcomes, are well known and are considered in Chapter 1.[30] The potential for residual confounding is further increased if social class groups are 'lumped', for example into manual and non-manual groups, as is common in many studies. Classifications based on SES proxies such as 'employed versus unemployed' and 'mother living versus not living with infant's father', though likely to identify materially deprived groups, tend to conceal the socioeconomic heterogeneity of the groups.[20,31]

The increased potential for residual confounding in studies of pregnancy and early childhood outcomes is confirmed by the evidence that within each social group smoking in pregnancy picks out those mothers with the lowest income, those least likely to own their own house, and length of time in poverty.[18,32] Thus smoking itself acts as a measure of intra-group or intra-class deprivation, increasing its apparent independent effects when inadequate SES classifications are used.

A further methodological problem is the introduction of systematic bias either by matching controls for SES-related factors or using outcome measures standardised for SES-related factors. Matching of controls for birth weight or local area of residence when studying outcomes in infancy, such as SIDS, incorporates a control for SES which will minimise the SES differential noted by the study and allow the effects attributable to other variables, such as smoking, to appear more powerful.[31,33] The same result will be achieved if the outcome under study is corrected for a factor which is itself SES-related.

In an otherwise well-designed study, Brooke and co-workers conclude that smoking is the single most important risk factor in the reduction of birth weight.[12] However, the main outcome was birth weight corrected for maternal height, itself strongly correlated with SES.

The emphasis in research on health-related behaviour influences the focus of study analysis.[2] A study of hospital admission in childhood reported an increased risk of admission for respiratory and other causes in children exposed to parental smoking, but re-analysis of the data shows that the risk of admission for low income groups was higher than that for the children of smokers.[34,28]

The apparent dose-related effect of maternal smoking on SIDS may also be spurious. Quantity of cigarettes smoked by mothers in pregnancy and by parents once the infant is born is strongly related to deprivation, with the heavy smokers clustering among the most deprived.[17,18] The conclusion that increasing deprivation is associated with increasing risk of SIDS and that smoking is acting as a marker of deprivation and a confounder is equally plausible, and is lent support by data from a major US study summarised in Table 8.3.

Data linking income and SIDS from the NICHD SIDS Cooperative Epidemiology Study (*see* Table 8.3) were adjusted for confounding variables, including smoking and 'race'. Income continued to be a powerful risk factor after adjusting for confounders.[35] Similar findings were reported from the large case–control study of sudden unexpected death in infancy, forming part of the Confidential Enquiry into Stillbirths and Deaths in Infancy (CESDI),[36] in which low income and receipt of state benefits retained an independent effect on sudden unexpected death, after controlling for smoking and other variables. The authors, in reporting the results in a subsequent paper, acknowledge this independent effect but choose to classify these SES measures as 'unmodifiable' factors, enabling them to continue to insist that behavioural as opposed to structural interventions are needed to further reduce the incidence of sudden unexpected deaths.[37]

In summary, passive smoking in pregnancy and in early childhood is likely to be detrimental to the health of the parent

Table 8.3   'Race' and average income per person (AIP) adjusted odds ratios for five commonly studied risk factors for sudden infant death syndrome. (Source [35] p. 225)

	Odds ratio		
Factor/Race	Low AIP	Medium AIP	High AIP
Maternal age			
Non-Black*	1.5	1.3	3.9
Black	1.6	4.9	3.4
Parity			
Non-Black	1.7	1.4	2.2
Black*	2.5	3.3	1.6
Smoking			
Non-Black*	3.2	2.7	1.8
Black*	3.3	3.5	9.3
Moved			
Non-Black*	1.7	1.7	2.0
Black*	1.7	2.6	6.0
Birth length			
Non-Black*	2.5	5.1	1.7
Black*	4.6	1.9	1.8

* Odds ratios significantly different across AIP strata, $P < 0.05$.

and the child. However, it is unlikely to account for the SES differentials in child health outcomes. There is very powerful evidence that in periods and countries where smoking was or is rare among women, SES differentials were and are present. Rather than accounting for child health inequalities, smoking seems to have become one of the factors in the pathways by which complex SES factors influence health outcomes (*see* Chapter 9).

Nutrition and child health

With the exception of specific conditions such as iron-deficiency anaemia and dental caries, there is little hard evidence linking nutritional variables to health outcomes in developed countries with a relative abundance of food.[38,39] Dietary recommendations vary between countries and within countries over time.[38]

For example, UK recommended intakes of daily nutrients have changed from the more prescriptive RDI (recommended daily intake) and RDA (recommended daily amount) to the more flexible EAR (estimate of average requirement), RNI (reference nutrient intake) and LRNI (lower reference nutrient intake) in recognition of the wide range of requirement for 'normal' growth and development.[38]

Dietary recommendations for children, produced by the UK Committee on Medical Aspects of Food Policy (COMA) are based on two premises: first, calorie-sufficient, balanced dietary intake (including fat, protein and carbohydrate, vitamins and essential and trace elements)[40] thought to ensure optimum growth at various ages; second, a diet which is thought to be optimal for adult health and contribute to the prevention of hypertension, heart disease and obesity. Neither premise is based on precise data and both have to take account of many variables, including cultural differences in diet and differences in the availability of various foods. Notwithstanding these limitations, the recommendations have been incorporated into health promotion material and form the standard against which the appropriateness of diets is measured.[41] In the UK, the National Advisory Council on Nutritional Education (NACNE) concluded in their 1983 report that there is strong evidence for dietary links with, among others, coronary heart disease, obesity, diabetes and hypertension, and consumption of animal fats, sugar and salt should be reduced and the intake of fibre, fresh fruit and polyunsaturated fats increased.[42]

Though food is now generally plentiful in developed countries compared with less developed countries (*see* Chapter 5) and the developed countries in the 19th century (*see* Chapter 4), marked social class differences in diet have been noted (Table 8.4).[43]

When considered in terms of recommended healthy diets such as that proposed by the NACNE, low income families in the UK consume a less healthy diet than higher income families: their diet is lower in essential nutrients such as calcium, iron, magnesium, folate and vitamin C, and new nutritional knowledge on the protective role of antioxidants and other dietary factors suggests that there is scope for health gain if a diet rich

Table 8.4 Food and nutrients with higher and lower consumption levels in low income families in 1995. (Source [43] p. 123)

Data source	Reference	Comparison	Higher in low income/ socio-economic group	Lower in low income/ socio-economic group
National Food Survey (1995)	MAFF (1996)	Income Group A (high) versus Income Group D and E2 (low)	*Foods:* White bread Full-fat milk Carcase meat and meat products Eggs Total fats Sugar Potatoes Tea *Nutrients (as % DRV):* Retinol equivalents Vitamin D Sodium Thiamin Vitamin B$_6$	Reduced-fat milk Cheese Poultry Fish Fresh green vegetables Other fresh vegetables Fruit Brown and wholemeal bread Breakfast cereals Coffee Soft drinks Alcoholic beverages Confectionery Magnesium Vitamin C

Table 8.4 Continued

Data source	Reference	Comparison	Higher in low income/ socio-economic group	Lower in low income/ socio-economic group
Infants up to 1 year	Martin and White (1988) Mills and Tyler (1992)	Social class I versus IV + V Socio-economic groups ABC1 versus C2DE	*Foods:* Infant formulas Potatoes Biscuits Confectionery Squashes and soft drinks *Nutrients:* Saturated fatty acids Dietary cholesterol	Breast milk Cow's milk and milk products Fruit Carotene Vitamin C
Toddlers 1½–4½ years	Gregory *et al.* (1995)	Social class I, II, IIIN (non-manual) versus IIIM, IV, V (manual) Not in receipt of benefit versus in receipt of benefit	*Foods:* White bread Non-high fibre breakfast cereal Milk puddings Skimmed milk Margarine (non-PUFA) Coated chicken Burgers and kebabs Meat pies and pastries	Pizza Wholewheat/soft grain bread Biscuits and fruit pies Sponge puddings Semi-skimmed milk Infant formula Cottage cheese Lamb, chicken, turkey, liver Raw and salad vegetables

continued overleaf

Table 8.4 Continued

Data source	Reference	Comparison	Higher in low income/ socio-economic group	Lower in low income/ socio-economic group
			Chips and crisps	Fresh vegetables
			Sugar	Fruit
			Chocolate and confectionery	Fruit juice
			Soft and alcoholic beverages	Commercial infant drinks
			Tea and coffee	
			Nutrients:	
			Energy (lone-parent children)	Non-starch polysaccharides
			Non-milk extrinsic sugar	β-carotene equivalents
			Starch	Vitamin C
			Sodium	Iron
				Calcium
				Iodine

Table 8.4 Continued

Data source	Reference	Comparison	Higher in low income/ socio-economic group	Lower in low income/ socio-economic group
Schoolchildren 10–15 years	Wenlock et al. (1986) DHSS (1989)	Social class I versus V Not in receipt of supplementary benefit versus in receipt of benefit Father employed versus unemployed	*Foods:* Total bread White bread Eggs Total potato Chips Baked beans (older children) Sugar *Nutrients:*	Milk Carcass meat Chicken Citrus fruit Apples and pears Carotene Vitamin C
Adults 16–64 years	Gregory et al. (1990) MAFF (1994)	Social classes I + II versus IV + V	*Foods:* White bread Soft margarine Chips Total potatoes Sugar	High fibre breakfast cereal Semi-skimmed milk Salad vegetables Total fruit Apples and pears Chocolate Wine, fortified wine and spirits

continued overleaf

Table 8.4 Continued

Data source	Reference	Comparison	Higher in low income/ socio-economic group	Lower in low income/ socio-economic group
			Nutrients:	Calcium Iron β-carotene Vitamin C Vitamin E

References:
- Gregory J, Collins DL, Davies PSW et al. (1995) National Diet and Nutrition Survey: children aged 1½ to 4½ years. HMSO, London.
- Gregory J, Foster K, Tyler H et al. (1990) The Dietary and Nutritional Survey of British Adults. HMSO, London.
- MAFF (Ministry of Agriculture, Fisheries and Food) (1996) National Food Survey 1995. HMSO, London.
- Martin J and White A (1988) Infant Feeding 1985. HMSO, London.
- Mills A and Tyler H (1992) Food and Nutrient Intakes of British Infants Aged 6–12 Months. HMSO, London.
- Wenlock RW, Disselduff MM and Skinner RK (1986) The Diets of British Schoolchildren: preliminary report. HMSO, London.

in vegetables, fruit, unrefined cereals, fish and quality vegetable oils were more accessible to them.[44]

It has been suggested that these dietary differences may partially explain health inequalities in infancy, childhood and later adult life. The causal debate has focused on the reasons for the dietary differences. The behavioural school maintains that lack of knowledge and failure to use resources properly explains the social class gradient in nutritional intakes. Ann Widdecombe, at the time a junior social security minister in the UK Government, in response to a survey by the UK-based charity, National Children's Homes, showing nutritional problems among low income families (*see* below), is quoted as saying:

> *I have to say that if I was trying to buy nutritional foods at good value, probably the last place I'd be going is the supermarket and certainly the last thing I'd be doing is looking among the ready-made foods … . How about a proper market where the food is at the cheapest?*[45,46]

This assumption that lack of knowledge and injudicious buying are at the root of the differences in food consumption between social groups has influenced much of the health promotion material related to nutrition.[47] This is reflected in socio-medical research conclusions – for example, Haste and co-workers, reporting their detailed study of social determinants of nutrient intake in pregnancy, show a strong correlation of low income with mean energy intakes of less than 80% of the RDI for pregnancy, but conclude that:

> *Specifically targeting pregnant women who are smokers, accommodation renters [a proxy for low income] and/or of minimum education (or perhaps low social class where other information is not available) for dietary advice would be appropriate, as well as offering advice on giving up smoking.*[32]

The following are implicit in the conclusions and recommendations of the behavioural school:

- All sections of the population have the same choices related to diet and food consumption.

- Lack of knowledge is the main determinant of poor dietary intake in low income families.

- Dietary education is likely to be the most effective health and social policy response.

Whereas dietary education and advice, which is sensitive to social context and has the active cooperation of the target group, has been shown to influence family diets, a wealth of evidence challenges the assumptions of free choice and lack of knowledge as the main determinant of unhealthy eating among the poor.[41,48,49]

Free choice assumes equality of access to healthy foods. In less developed countries a high percentage of household income spent on food is a powerful marker of poverty (*see* Chapter 5, p. 117).[50] Families in the lowest income decile in the UK in 1995–96 spent 30% of their income on food compared with only 18% for families in the highest income decile.[43] Families dependent on state benefits in the 1991 NCH Nutrition Survey spent over 35% of their household income on food.[45] However, despite a far higher proportion of expenditure on food, low income families had far less money in absolute terms to spend on food – in 1995–96, the comparative figures were an average of £17 per person for low income families and £29 per person for high income families.[43]

These differences in absolute amount of income available for food expenditure would be less important if healthy food were cheap and readily accessible without expensive transport.[43] However, healthy foods are more expensive and the cost per calorie is higher.[51] Table 8.5 compares the cost per 100 kcal of various food items.

The price of healthy foods is not only higher but the trend is towards an increasing price disparity between healthy and unhealthy foods (*see* Table 8.6).[52]

Table 8.5   Cost per 100 kcal of 'healthy' and 'unhealthy' foods in the UK in the 1980s. (Source [51])

	Cost (pence)/100 kcal
Lean beef	40
Cod fillet	50
Lean pork	23
Chicken leg	18
Meat pies	7
Sausages	6
Tomatoes	70
Cabbage	15
Potatoes	6
Chips	6
Crisps	9
Oranges	25
Apples	14
Mars Bar	8
Fruit juice	20
Cola drink	16
Lard	1
Sugar	2
White bread	2
Wholemeal bread	3

Table 8.6   Increases in food prices in the UK, 1982–86 – 'healthy' versus 'unhealthy' foods. (Source [52])

Healthy foods	%	Less healthy foods	%
Wholemeal bread	17	White bread	15
Green vegetables	17–51	Biscuits	19
Root vegetables	29–37	Sugar	13
Salad vegetables	22–42	Bacon	13
Fresh fruit	16–45	Sausages	13
Poultry	26	Whole milk	17
Fish	44	Butter	9

The above figures are taken from the UK; even in countries such as Spain, with a tradition of higher intake of fresh fruit and vegetables, healthy foods cost more and there is a tendency for healthy foods to be more expensive in the same super-market chain in poor compared with better off areas.[53] The same tendency for healthy foods to be more expensive in poorer areas has been demonstrated in a Scottish study.[54]

The nutritional restrictions imposed on families by inadequate income make it impossible to consume a healthy diet. A diet meeting the NACNE dietary requirements costs 35% more than the average amount spent by low income families on food.[43] Lobstein calculated that, in 1988, families dependent on state benefit had on average 2–3 pence per 100 kcal to spend on food for children in order to reach recommended daily calorie requirements of 1550 for small children and 2400 for older children.[51] Based on his cost per 100 kcal figures (Table 8.5), he comments that 'to stick rigidly to under 3p per 100 kcal implies a 19th-century diet of bread and dripping [equivalent to lard] and sweetened tea'.

Far from being able to afford a healthy diet, many members of low income families frequently go without any food, healthy or unhealthy.[55,56] Children are less likely to go without food as they are protected by their mothers, who are the family members most likely to manage without food; however, in the NCH survey, 10% of children surveyed had gone hungry during the preceding month because of lack of money.[45,57]

Dowler and Calvert, in their study of nutrition in lone-parent families in London, show a strong correlation between income level, as defined by a 'poverty index', and adequacy of nutrient intake which was independent of parental smoking. The correlation is shown in Figure 8.2.[57]

Lack of nutritional knowledge among the poor has also been challenged. UK studies have failed to show any major differences in knowledge between low and high income mothers, and low income mothers aspire to a healthy diet for their children as much as high income mothers.[45,58] There is some evidence that mothers from deprived areas, whilst understanding the basics of healthy eating, have more difficulty than their more privileged peers in understanding how to implement their knowledge.[41] However, the same publication acknowledges that the main problem seems to be a reluctance to try new foods unless they are offered free of charge. Other studies

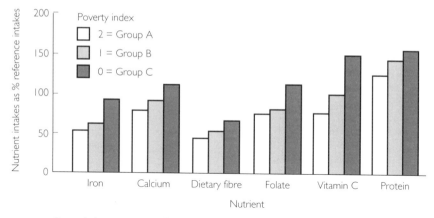

Group A: long-term unemployed council tenants, no holiday and whose rent or fuel is automatically deducted from their benefit or on a key metre
Group B: either unemployed council tenants or with fuel/rent deductions
Group C: neither category

Figure 8.2   Adequacy of lone-parents' nutrient intake from weighted food survey. (Source [57])

have demonstrated how difficult it is for families on low incomes to experiment with new foods, as rejection would lead to waste of scarce resources and family members would have to go hungry.[57]

Since the early 1980s eating patterns have changed in both high and low income groups, with a general move towards more healthy eating suggesting that low income families, despite the constraints of lack of money, are responding to the health education messages.[52] As Table 8.7 shows, low income families spend a larger proportion of their limited income on foods recommended as healthy than high income families.

In summary, there is little to support the assumptions underlying the behavioural explanations for inadequate nutrition among poor families; income and not lack of knowledge seems to be the main determinant of poor dietary intake in low income families. Choice without adequate income is an illusion. Structural explanations are able to account much more convincingly for the observed differences in diet between social groups. Not only are behavioural explanations unable to account

Table 8.7   Percentage of income spent on food in high and low income families. (Source [51])

	High income household (£)	Low income household (£)		% difference between high and low income household
		with earner	without earner	
Energy (kcal)	170.3	230	221	35%
Protein (g)	5.8	7.6	7.2	31%
Fat (g)	7.9	10.72	10.2	35%
Carbohydrate (g)	20.2	27.7	26.7	38%
Calcium (g)	75	98	93	30%
Iron (mg)	0.97	1.2	1.2	24%
Thiamin (mg)	0.11	0.15	0.14	36%
Riboflavin (mg)	0.15	0.19	0.18	27%
Niacin (mg)	2.4	3.0	2.8	25%
Vitamin C (mg)	6.6	5.6	5.6	15%
Vitamin A (mg)	98.6	143	142	45%
Vitamin D (mg)	0.26	0.34	0.35	31%
Weekly amount spent	£11.86	£8.58	£9.71	

for the observed differences in diet between social groups, but when adopted by professionals they are likely to undermine the efforts of women in low income families to provide adequate nutrition for their children. As Travers suggests:

> As long as professional practice continues to place primary emphasis on changing individuals without consideration of the context within which they work, the potential remains high for victim blaming on the part of the professionals, and guilt on the part of the individual who is unable to live up to expectations. ([59] p. 551)

Hygiene and child health in less developed countries and in developed countries in the 19th and early 20th centuries

Even in settings where absolute poverty exists, there are conflicting explanations for socio-economic differences in child health outcomes. This aspect of the causal debate is addressed in detail in Chapter 5 (p. 123) but is summarised here. Behavioural explanations broadly focus on hygiene practices and lack of maternal knowledge, as well as cultural practices influencing child rearing and food preparation and consumption as the main determinants of adverse child health outcomes. Structural explanations stress the socio-economic, societal and environmental influences on families which modify and, to some extent, determine cultural patterns of behaviour and individual knowledge and hygiene practices.

Water- and airborne diseases are responsible for a large part of the child mortality and morbidity in less developed countries (*see* Chapter 5) and in developed countries in the 19th and early 20th centuries (*see* Chapter 4, p. 91). In contrast to the debate in developed countries, explanations for the high prevalence of these diseases and their concentration among the poor in less developed countries have focused on hygiene, cultural practices, family size, overcrowding, maternal education, water availability and living conditions. The health-related behaviours, such as smoking, which have dominated the causal debate in developed countries, have found little place so far in relation to developing countries and, by women at least, were not practised by the poor in today's developed countries in the 19th and early 20th centuries. In the same way as advocates of behavioural explanations for inequalities in present-day developed countries, advocates of the behavioural school in less developed countries concentrate on the individual family, and usually the mother within that family. Differences in hygiene and knowledge as well as culturally determined practices are presented as the main explanations for adverse outcomes in early childhood.[60,61] Similar explanations were advanced by some researchers for the differences in outcomes in today's developed countries in the 19th century.[62] In the UK, alarm was expressed in the early part of the 20th century at the poor health of young military conscripts and enquiries were undertaken by government to ascertain the reasons. Some of the explanations advanced by health professionals at the time are revealing:

> *The girls ... have no sort of sense of duty; not the slightest. It is only amusement and pleasure with them. The last thing they think of is duty, and therefore, they do not trouble to cook or get up in the morning, and the children go to school without breakfast because the woman is too idle to get up ... she is utterly indifferent.* (Evidence by a voluntary health visitor to the Inter-Departmental Committee on Physical Deterioration, 1904.[63])

> *It is ignorance and carelessness of mothers that directly cause a large proportion of infant mortality .... What is needed is training in those arts of domestic management of which compulsory education has deprived the girls of the artisan classes.* (Taken from George Newman *Infant Mortality: A Social Problem*, 1906.[63])

These views of the poor at home were echoed in the attitudes to overt poverty in the colonies. The following quote is taken from Webster and records the attitude of the Sanitary Commission in the French North African port of Dakar to the living conditions of the Africans during an outbreak of plague:

> *... the transfer of the native population which takes pleasure in a deep-rooted and incurable filthiness, to a place far from the city, and the destruction or demolition of all shacks and huts, as the only measure able to stop the spread of the current epidemic.* ([62] p. 84)

The following assumptions are implicit in the conclusions and recommendations of the behavioural school in relation to health outcomes in less developed countries and historically in today's developed countries:

- Personal hygiene and knowledge are the main determinants of child health differences.

- Culturally determined factors also play an important role, independent of SES.

- Policies which increase knowledge and change individual behaviour are the key to change in adverse childhood outcomes.

These assumptions are challenged by the structural school on the basis that individual behavioural and cultural factors are themselves closely linked to SES. For example, maternal education, universally accepted as an important determinant of child health outcomes in less developed countries, is itself positively correlated with higher SES in less developed countries (see Chapter 5), and the power of its effect can be modified by governments through health and social policies.[64,65] Personal hygiene is also strongly influenced by socio-economic resources which determine access to sanitation and clean water as well as influencing the capacity of a mother to maintain standards against the odds of adverse environmental conditions (see Chapter 4).

Many of the studies on which the behavioural assumptions are based have been challenged (see Chapter 4). Some of the studies have been conducted in single villages where the socio-economic spectrum is small and the major differences between rich and poor cannot be examined; others have used SES measures which are inappropriately defined and insensitive to variations among rural families.[66] Millard has also criticised the focus on infant mortality rather than child mortality (under-five mortality) on the basis that:

> It can result in a biased view of the demography of less developed countries, because infant mortality includes only an arbitrary segment of a continuous phenomenon extending well beyond the first year of life. ([66] p. 590)

Structural explanations for child health inequalities, in all three of the specific situations examined above, are thus more robust. Behavioural factors, such as smoking, diet and hygiene, have a role but they cannot explain the extent of differences between social groups, and are themselves closely SES correlated and form part of the complex pathways by which socio-economic and socio-cultural factors influence health (*see* Chapter 9).

Summary

1   The causal debate is part of a wider political debate centring on the roles and responsibilities of individuals and societies in ensuring their health and welfare.

2   Behavioural explanations for health inequalities are currently dominant and have a powerful influence on health and social policy.

3   Particular methodological interpretations of socio-medical research data have contributed to the dominance of behavioural explanations and there is an urgent need for review of research methodology in the area of socio-medical research.

4   Structural explanations for health inequalities are more consistent with available evidence and, in particular, the historical and international evidence presented in the previous section of this book.

References

1   Townsend P and Davidson N (1982) *Inequalities in Health: The Black Report*. Penguin, Harmondsworth.

2   Smith GD, Blane D and Bartley M (1994) Explanations of socio-economic differences in mortality: evidence from Britain and elsewhere. *Eur. J. Public Health*. **131**:131–44.

3   Power C, Manor O and Fox J (1991) Health and social inequality in Europe. *BMJ*. **308**:1153–6.

4   Blane D, Power C and Bartley M (1996) Illness behaviour and the measurement of class differentials in morbidity. *J. Roy. Stat. Soc.* **Series A**. **159**:77–92.

5   Macintyre S (1986) The patterning of health by social position in contemporary Britain: directions for sociological research. *Soc. Sci. Med.* **23**:393–415.

6   Royal College of Physicians of London (1992) *Smoking and the Young: A Report of a Working Party of the RCP*. RCP, London.

7   Department of Health (1992) *The Health of the Nation: A Strategy for Health in England*. HMSO, London.

8   Department of Health (1998*)* Independent inquiry into inequalities in health (The Acheson Report). The Stationery Office, London.

9   United Nations Development Programme (1994) *Human Development Report*. UNDP and Oxford University Press, New York.

10 Himmelberger D, Brown B and Cohen E (1978) Cigarette smoking during pregnancy and the occurrence of spontaneous abortion and congenital abnormality. *Am. J. Epidemiol.* **108**:470–9.

11 Comstock GW, Shah FK, Meyer MB *et al.* (1971) Low birth weight and neonatal mortality related to maternal smoking and socioeconomic status. *Am. J. Obstet. Gynecol.* **111**:53–9.

12 Brooke OG, Anderson HR, Bland JM *et al.* (1989) The effects on birth weight of smoking, alcohol, caffeine, socioeconomic factors and psychosocial stress. *BMJ*. **298**:795–801.

13 Chen Y, Li W and Yu S (1986) Influence of passive smoking on admissions for respiratory illness in early childhood. *BMJ*. **293**:303–6.

14   Golding J (1997) Sudden infant death syndrome and parental smoking: a literature review. *Paediatr. Perinat. Epidemiol.* **11**:67–77.

15   Fogelman K (1980) Smoking in pregnancy and subsequent development of the child. *Child: Care, Health and Development.* **6**:233–49.

16   Conroy S and Smith M (1999) *Exploring Infant Health.* The Foundation for the Study of Infant Deaths, London.

17   Graham H (1993) *Smoking Among Working Class Women's Lives.* Harvester Wheatsheaf, Hemel Hempstead.

18   Graham H and Blackburn C (1998) The socio-economic patterning of health and smoking behaviour among mothers with young children on income support. *Sociol. Health and Illness.* **20**:215–40.

19   Nicholl J and O'Cathain A (1992) Smoking and the Sudden Infant Death Syndrome. In *Effects of Smoking on the Fetus, Neonate and Child* (eds D Poswillo and E Alberman). Oxford Medical Publications, Oxford.

20   Haglund B and Cnattingius S (1990) Cigarette smoking as a risk factor for sudden infant death syndrome: a population-based study. *Am. J. Public Health.* **80**:29–32.

21   Burton GJ (1992) The effects of maternal cigarette smoking on placental structure and function in mid to late gestation. In *Effects of Smoking on the Fetus, Neonate and Child* (eds D Poswillo and A Alberman). Oxford Medical Publications, Oxford.

22   Golding J, Fleming PJ and Parkes S (1992) Cot deaths and sleep position campaigns. *Lancet.* **339**:743–9.

23   Blackburn C and Graham H (1993) *Smoking Amongst Working Class Mothers – An Information Pack.* Department of Applied Social Studies, University of Warwick, Coventry.

24   Graham H (1987) Women's smoking and family health. *Soc. Sci. Med.* **25**:47–56.

25 Graham H (1996) Smoking prevalence among women in the European Community, 1950–1990. *Soc. Sci. Med.* **43**:243–54.

26 Ministerio de Sanidad y Consumo, Spain (1987) *National Smoking Survey.* Ministerio de Sanidad y Consumo, Madrid.

27 Griva E, Tsirka A, Lolis D *et al.* (1987) *Frequency of Smoking in Pregnant Women.* 25th National Paediatric Conference, Patra, Greece (Abstract No. 54).

28 Logan S and Spencer NJ (1996) Smoking and other health-related behaviour in the social and environmental context. *Arch. Dis. Child.* **74**:716–9.

29 Smith GD and Phillips AN (1992) Confounding in epidemiological studies: why 'independent' effects may not be all they seem. *BMJ.* **305**:757–9.

30 Oakley A, Rigby AS and Hickey D (1993) Women and children last? Class, health and the role of maternal and child health services. *Eur. J. Public Health.* **3**:220–6.

31 Gilbert R, Rudd P and Berry PJ (1992) Combined effects of infection and heavy wrapping in the risk of sudden unexpected infant death. *Arch. Dis. Child.* **67**:171–7.

32 Haste FM, Brooke OE, Anderson HR *et al.* (1990) Social determinants of nutrient intake in smokers and non-smokers during pregnancy. *J. Epidemiol. Community Health.* **44**: 205–9.

33 Kraus AS, Steele RA, Thompson MG *et al.* (1971) Further epidemiologic observation on sudden unexpected death in infancy in Ontario. *Can. J. Public Health.* **62**:210–18.

34 Harlap S and Davies A (1974) Infant admissions to hospital and maternal smoking. *Lancet.* **i**:529–32.

35 Kraus JF, Petersen DR, Standfast SJ *et al.* (1988) The relationship of socioeconomic status and sudden infant death syndrome: confounding or effect modifier. In *Sudden*

Infant Death Syndrome: Risk Factors and Basic Mechanisms (eds RM Harper and HJ Hoffman). PMA Publishing Corp., New York.

36 Department of Health (1996) *Confidential Enquiry into Stillbirths and Deaths in Infancy: 3rd Annual Report, 1st January–31st December, 1994*. Department of Health, London.

37 Blair PS, Fleming PJ, Bacon C *et al.* (1996) Smoking and the sudden infant death syndrome: results from a case–control study for the Confidential Enquiry into Stillbirths and Deaths in Infancy. *BMJ*. 313:195–9.

38 Aukett MA and Wharton BA (1995) Suboptimal nutrition. In *Social Paediatrics* (eds B Lindstrom and NJ Spencer). Oxford University Press, Oxford.

39 Carmichael CL, Rugg-Gun AJ and Ferrell RS (1989) The relationship between fluoridation, social class and caries experience in 5-year old children in Newcastle and Northumberland. *Br. Dent. J.* 167:57–61.

40 Department of Health and Social Security (DHSS) (1988) *Present-day Practice in Infant Feeding: Third Report*. Reports on Health and Social Subjects, No. 36. HMSO, London.

41 National Dairy Council (1993) *Nutrition and Low Income Families*. National Dairy Council Publication, London.

42 Health Education Council/National Advisory Committee on Nutrition Education (NACNE) (1983) *Proposals for Nutritional Guidelines in Britain: a Discussion Paper*. HMSO, London.

43 Nelson M (1999) Nutrition and health inequalities. In *Inequalities in Health* (eds D Gordon, M Shaw, D Dorling *et al.*). The Policy Press, University of Bristol, Bristol.

44 James JW, Nelson M, Ralph A *et al.* (1998) Socio-economic determinants of health: the contribution of nutrition to inequalities in health. *BMJ*. 316:308–9.

45 National Children's Homes (1991) *NCH Poverty and Nutrition Survey.* NCH, London.

46 Widdecombe A (1991) Comments in response to NCH Poverty and Nutrition Survey. *The Guardian*, 4th June, 1991.

47 Research Unit in Health and Behavioural Change (RUHBC) (1989) *Changing the Public Health*. Wiley, Chichester.

48 James J, Brown J, Douglas M *et al.* (1992) Improving the diet of under-fives in a deprived inner-city practice. *Health Trends*. **24**:161–4.

49 National Food Alliance (1994) *Food and Low Income: A Practical Guide*. National Food Alliance, London.

50 Grant J (1994) *The State of the World's Children*. Oxford University Press, New York.

51 Lobstein T (1988) Poor children and cheap calories. *Community Paediatric Group Newsletter* (in association with the British Paediatric Association). **Autumn**:4–5.

52 Blackburn C (1991) *Poverty and Health: Working with Families*. Open University Press, Milton Keynes.

53 Vanndrager L, Colomer C and Ashton J (1992) Inequalities in nutritional choice: a baseline study from Valencia. *Health Promotion Int*. **7**:109–17.

54 Sooman A, Macintyre S and Anderson A (1993) Scotland's health – a more difficult challenge for some? The price and availability of healthy foods in socially contrasting localities in the West of Scotland. *Health Bull*. **51**:276–84.

55 Lang T (1984) *Jam Tomorrow?* Food Policy Unit, Manchester Polytechnic, Manchester.

56 Cole-Hamilton I and Lang T (1986) *Tightening Belts: A Report of the Impact of Poverty on Food*. London Food Commission, London.

57   Dowler E and Calvert C (1995) *Nutrition and Diet in Lone-parent Families in London*. Family Policy Centre and the Joseph Rowntree Foundation, London.

58   Calnan M (1988) Food and health: a comparison of beliefs and practices in middle-class and working-class households. In *Readings in Medical Sociology* (eds S Cunningham-Birley and N McKegary). Tavistock, London.

59   Travers KD (1996) The social organization of nutritional inequalities. *Soc. Sci. Med.* **43**:543–53.

60   Moy RJD, Booth IW, Choto R-GAB *et al.* (1991) Risk factors for high diarrhoea frequency: a study in rural Zimbabwe. *Trans Roy. Soc. Trop. Med. Hyg.* **85**:814–18.

61   Stanton BF and Clemens JD (1987) An educational intervention for altering water sanitation behaviors to reduce childhood diarrhea in urban Bangladesh. II. A randomized trial to assess the impact of the intervention on hygiene behaviors and rates of diarrhea. *Am. J. Epidemiol.* **125**:292–301.

62   Webster C (ed.) (1993) *Caring for Health: History and Diversity*. Open University Press, Milton Keynes.

63   Smith D and Nicholson M (1992) Poverty and ill health: controversies past and present. *Proc. Roy. Coll. Physicians Edinburgh.* **22**:190–9.

64   Caldwell J and MacDonald P (1982) Influence of maternal education in infant and child mortality: levels and causes. *Health Policy Educ.* **2**:251–67.

65   Palloni A (1981) Mortality in Latin America: emerging patterns. *Popul. Dev. Rev.* **7**:623–48.

66   Millard AV (1985) Child mortality and economic variation among rural Mexican households. *Soc. Sci. Med.* **20**:589–99.

9

Mechanisms, causal models and pathways

Introduction

Despite the protracted nature of the causal debate, there has been little attention paid to the mechanisms by which poverty and low SES may influence health. Having concluded in the previous chapter that the behavioural explanations are inadequate to explain social gradients in child health, I explore possible mechanisms. Finally, alternative approaches to studying social gradients in health outcomes, which avoid some common methodological pitfalls and acknowledge the social context of health-related behaviour, are considered.

Mechanisms by which socio-economic status influences health

Previous chapters have established the strong link between socio-economic factors and child health, and the discussion shows that structural explanations are the most consistent with the findings from earlier historical periods in today's developed countries as well as present-day less developed and developed countries. However, socio-economic factors are mediated by many other factors and exploration of these mediators helps to validate and elucidate the links between SES and health outcomes.

Unemployment

In all societies and in all historical periods, except for privileged minorities who inherit or control financial resources and thus have no need to work, the availability of paid employment, or work in exchange for goods, has been linked with income and SES. Those without any or regular employment have tended to be at the lower end of the socio-economic spectrum. In less developed and developed countries, unemployment and underemployment are important determinants of poverty (*see* Chapter 2, p. 40). Recent research in developed countries has established the close links between unemployment and poor adult health outcomes.[1] Length of time unemployed is correlated with increased mortality: men who had been unemployed at the time of both the 1971 and 1981 Censuses had a standardised mortality ratio of 194 in the years between 1981 and 1992 compared with 83 for those employed at both Censuses and 127 for those unemployed at only one Census.[1] The sharp increases in unemployment in some developed countries in the 1980s, differentially affecting regions and localities, have contributed to the increasing disparity of health outcomes for all age groups.[2-4] Unemployment has disproportionately affected young adults and their families, contributing to the trend which has resulted in children becoming the largest group in poverty (*see* Chapter 2, p. 40). Though not themselves unemployed, the well-being and development of these children is threatened as much by the depression and stress experienced by their parents as by the resulting poverty and diminished access to the rich array of consumer goods passing across their television screens.[5,6]

Unemployment and underemployment have community as well as individual effects. Their concentration in some localities has created communities in which the majority of residents are without work and are dependent on state benefits.[1] For example, in Glasgow Springburn electoral ward in 1991, 47.2% of men aged 16–64 were unemployed (25.0%), permanently sick (15.2%), retired early (2.5%) or economically inactive for other reasons (4.4%).[1] Such communities suffer disproportionately from crime and vandalism and the collapse of infrastructure such as leisure facilities, healthcare provision and shops. Schools serving these areas tend to reflect the general level of deprivation and become 'sink' schools from which middle class parents remove their children. The cumulative effect is to further disadvantage children being brought up in these communities and to increase the prospect of them following their parents into, at best, low-paid precarious employment and, at worst, long-term unemployment. In the UK and USA these effects are exacerbated by racism, with the result that black children and young people suffer 'double jeopardy' (*see* Chapter 1, p. 5).

Debt, resources and fuel poverty

Closely linked with unemployment, underemployment and low income and survival in a consumerist society is the phenomenon of debt. A UK-based survey reported an increase in households living on credit since 1970, and those most dependent on, and in most trouble as a consequence of, credit were young families with children living on state benefits or low income.[7] There is also an increase in multiple debt, where money is owed to more than one creditor, and families on state benefit have been reported as typically having debts equivalent to four times their average family income.[8] For many low income families credit is used for necessities rather than for luxuries and the birth of a child tends to increase family expenditure and reduce earning capacity.[9] For most of these families debt is directly related to low income despite tight money management.[10]

Women and children are the most vulnerable to the effects of debt.[10] Women are more likely to take responsibility for the payment of bills, though they are less likely to have control of family finances.[8,10] They suffer guilt and feelings of failure such that the level of debt is often hidden from their partners.[8,10] When partners are aware of the level of debt, it is reported by mothers as a major source of conflict.[10] As considered above, women tend to protect their children and partners from the worst effects of low income and debt: they restrict their own diets and seek solace and relief in cigarette smoking to the detriment of their health.[8,11] Women are also vulnerable to imprisonment for non-payment of debts, particularly TV licence debt.[1] Children may also go without food but are most likely to suffer as a result of their mothers' depression and the conflict resulting from their parents' struggle to make ends meet.

A further consequence of the extremes of debt for low income families is disconnection or supply restriction of essential services such as electricity, gas and water. An increased number of families in the UK had their electricity and/or gas supply disconnected in the 1980s and early 1990s. Water privatisation in the UK has led to an increase in water charges and the introduction of water meters in many areas, with the result that increasing numbers of poor people have had their water disconnected (12 000 in England and Wales in 1993) or have had to reduce the amount of water used for bathing and washing. The effects of depriving families with children of heating fuel and water are likely to lead to increased susceptibility of children to respiratory and gastrointestinal illnesses.

Underpinning the increase in debt amongst low income families in the UK is the increase in income inequality in the last 20–30 years. Average real household disposable income, after the effects of inflation and taxes etc. have been removed, rose by 72% between 1961 and 1994.[1] This increase, however, has been unevenly spread throughout the population: the proportion of low income households has risen from one in ten in 1961 to one in five in 1990. For families with children the differential income changes have been even more striking: among large families with three children the poorest 10% were, on average, £625 poorer in 1995–96 than in 1979 whereas the richest 10% were a staggering £21 000 richer.[1]

Housing and the environment

Overcrowded, inadequate housing has been known for many years to have a detrimental effect on health (*see* also Chapters 4, 5 and 6).[12] In developed and less developed countries inadequate housing is strongly correlated with poverty and low income.[13] In the UK in 1986, 2.5 million dwellings were assessed as being in poor condition, of which 1 million were

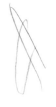

judged unfit for human habitation.[13] Many live in housing chronically affected by damp and mould – it has been estimated that 30% of all local authority housing (rented social housing) in the North of England and Scotland suffers some degree of damp, causing internal pollution.[12]

In less developed countries many children are without homes, living on the streets of the large cities.[14] In developed countries there has been a marked increase in homelessness: in 1992, nearly 170 000 households, most of which included children, were statutorily homeless in Britain.[15] Such households are universally poor and the majority dependent on state benefits. The increase in homelessness in recent years among families with young children can be directly related in the UK to government policy, and specifically 'the destruction of housing as a public service'.[15] The lack of affordable housing means that families are housed in multiple-occupation hotels and 'bed and breakfast' accommodation, which are unsuitable and dangerous for young children as well as being highly expensive. Now and in the past, poor families have been obliged to live in the least desirable areas whilst those with more financial resources have been able to choose more healthy environments. In the major cities of the less developed countries, slum housing tends to be concentrated in areas with major environmental hazards.[16] Cities in developed countries have similar concentrations of poor families in areas of high pollution, overcrowding and poor-quality services frequently close to major roads. These concentrations of poor housing (sometimes called 'inner-city areas', though many lie on the outskirts of cities) tend to house the poorest families. Crime, unemployment, drug and substance abuse, family violence and educational underachievement are prevalent in these areas, creating a poor and threatening environment for child rearing.[17,18]

In addition to the structural and environmental hazards of poor areas, services tend to be inadequate or of poor quality with limited public transport, low-quality, expensive food shops and few leisure facilities, especially for families and the young. These factors limit the ability of the poor to access the social and cultural life enjoyed by their fellow citizens, resulting in social exclusion. The adverse environmental conditions associated with poor neighbourhoods, such as proximity to main roads, poor amenities, lack of play areas and poor structural condition of housing, also make children more vulnerable to accidents.[19]

Thus, the structural integrity of housing and the environment in which the housing is situated have both a direct and an indirect effect on child and family health, causing physical and psychological morbidity.[20–22]

Nutrition

The relation of nutrition to child health was considered in detail in Chapter 8 (p. 218) as part of the causal debate. There is general agreement that nutrition is important to child health and that undernutrition is associated with increased mortality and morbidity in less developed countries (*see* Chapter 5). McKeown and others (*see* Chapter 4) have argued that the major decline in mortality in the developed countries was associated with improvements in nutrition and, as considered in Chapter 4 (p. 94), there is strong evidence for links between undernutrition and adverse child health outcomes in 19th-century Europe.

Nutrition insufficiency is prevalent in developed countries today. It has been estimated that 8% of US children less than eight years of age (4 million) experience prolonged periodic food insufficiency and hunger each year, with a further 10 million at risk of hunger.[23] Hunger and food insufficiency are strongly correlated with behavioural, emotional and academic problems.[23] Optimal nutrition seems to be important for the health and well-being of the embryo, the fetus and the growing child.[24–26] There is good evidence that women in low income groups are less well nourished before and during pregnancy, contributing to higher levels of adverse pregnancy outcomes. Children from low income families tend to have a relatively poor diet.[27] It is likely that there are inter-generational effects associated with poor nutrition in developed countries, though more subtle than those seen in less developed countries (*see* Chapter 5). A review of the data from the Dutch Hunger Winter of 1944–45 suggests that the pregnancies of women from the historically privileged region most affected by the famine were protected from its worst effects by their relative wealth and good nutritional status preceding the famine.[28] The author argues that optimal nutrition across generations acts as a protective factor against adverse events and that the reverse is also likely to be true – suboptimal nutrition increases vulnerability.

Education

There are well-established links between parental education levels and health outcomes for their children in both developed and less developed countries.[29,30] The relation of maternal education to child health is particularly strong.[31] As considered in Chapter 5 (p. 104), those poor countries which are 'high' health achievers have succeeded, in part, by achieving higher levels of female literacy.

Low levels of education are strongly correlated with SES in developed and less developed countries, partly as a result of the link between higher qualification and higher pay but also the exclusion of the poor from education opportunities. The link is so close that education levels are often used as SES proxies in socio-medical studies.

It also appears that poverty exerts a negative influence on the developmental and intellectual progress of children, independent of the educational level of their parents.[32] Parental depression and loss of self-esteem resulting from the privations of poverty have been shown to directly affect the developmental progress of children and the parenting strategies used.[32,33]

Poverty itself also seems to increase the chances of children suffering loss of self-esteem and mental disorders such as depression.[34,35] Poverty's influence on child development is also mediated through nutrition: iron-deficiency anaemia, the commonest nutritional deficiency in childhood, is associated with impaired development, and suboptimal maternal nutrition before and during pregnancy may directly influence embryonic and fetal brain growth and possibly intellectual capacity.[22,36] As considered above, hunger and food insufficiency may also be negatively correlated with academic achievement.[23]

Education not only implies greater earning capacity but enhances self-esteem and confidence, both of which are important in child rearing. Parents with low educational levels are less likely to challenge professional judgements or decisions related to the health of their children; the results of this powerlessness are seen in the studies of unexpected death in infancy, which have demonstrated the difficulty parents have in acting on their own judgement that their child is ill when professionals have dismissed their concerns.[37] Education confers power not just in the job market but also in the business of daily living.

However, just as with housing, unemployment and the environment, education is not a matter of individual choice and is broadly dependent on societal provision of, and commitment to, universal education. Most developed countries are characerised by high levels of literacy but there are marked variations in the extent to which educational provision is truly universal and in the priority given to education.[38] Education in less developed countries has suffered in the same way as health provision from financial constraints imposed by economic structural adjustment programmes supported by the IMF and the World Bank.[14,39]

Psychosocial effects, social exclusion and powerlessness

The positive correlation between more equitable income distribution and improved national mortality rates and life expectancy has been demonstrated in developed and less developed countries.[38,40,41] Wilkinson argues that this is unlikely to be due to absolute levels of income and better individual salary levels, but rather to improved social cohesion, with fewer people excluded from the mainstream of community life. He further postulates a broader influence on the health of the whole community: if there are high levels of social exclusion, as in the UK and USA, the well-being of the whole society is compromised, with adverse effects on health outcomes for the privileged as well as the disadvantaged.[40]

In exploring the mechanisms by which income maldistribution affects health, Wilkinson argues:

> *If circumstances impact on health less of their own accord than through a comparative process, this suggests that psychosocially mediated effects may be crucial. To give an example, attempts to account for the ill health associated with damp housing in terms of the direct effects of dampness have only been able to account for a very small part of the problem. While it was successfully demonstrated that the presence of mould spores in the air was responsible for some increase in rates of respiratory illness, most of the excess morbidity escapes this kind of analysis.[42] If the link with relative poverty implies what I have suggested, then what people feel about their housing, their financial and social circumstances is likely to be more important than their objective conditions.* ([43] p. 5)

These psychosocially-mediated effects are likely to manifest through lack of self-esteem and feelings of powerlessness. There is evidence linking these feelings with relative poverty and health outcomes for children as well as evidence for improvements in self-esteem and child rearing practices with improvements in SES.[32,44] Social exclusion appears to be closely related to increased levels of stress and impaired social support mechanisms.[33] All have been associated with poor health outcomes, particularly for women and children.[21,45]

In this context, it is worth giving brief consideration to the concepts of 'parenting failure' or not 'good enough' parenting,[46] often the focus of child protection work, and 'maternal incompetence/inefficiency', previously an accepted reason for poor infant health outcomes which remains a commonly held, though not explicitly stated, explanation for childhood illness and health-related problems. As the quotes from the beginning of the 20th century show (Chapter 8, p. 232), failings of individual mothers and their perceived indifference to the welfare of their children were seen as the main determinant of poor infant health. Later researchers utilised measures of maternal incompetence/inefficiency based on professional assessments of the child's personal hygiene, the state of the home (i.e. its cleanliness), the child's diet and the attitude of the mother to the child and, in one case, whether the child's shoe size was appropriate.[47,48] As with the concept of parenting failure in current child protection practice, these measures are divorced from social conditions and were applied with little recognition of the socially determined processes which underlie child caring and child rearing, and it is not surprising that the mothers judged 'incompetent' by these measures tended to live in conditions of material poverty and overcrowding.[47,49]

Social exclusion, powerlessness, loss of self-esteem, maternal depression and lack of supportive relationships and social support are all likely to contribute, along with poor physical living conditions and limited financial resources, to poor levels of hygiene, poor diet and home cleanliness, as well as having a direct effect on the parenting strategies used in child rearing.[32,50]

Social support and social capital

Social support, defined as 'resources provided by other persons', has been shown to influence health through a range of mechanisms – improving mental health and physical morbidity as well as influencing mortality.[51] The evidence linking lower socio-economic status with lower levels of social support is patchy and contradictory but there is good evidence that individuals in higher social groups enjoy more extensive and more confiding social networks.[51] At a societal level, the term 'social capital' has been coined to describe those features of social organisation, such as civic participation, norms of reciprocity and trust in others, that facilitate cooperation for mutual benefit.[52] This can be conceived of as social support at a societal level. Social capital seems to be positively correlated with improved levels of health and lower mortality rates.[40,52] More equitable income distribution is associated with increased social capital,[52] and is reported to be more closely correlated with improvements in under-five mortality rates than absolute income in Taiwan.[53]

Service access, availability and use

Tudor Hart argued that health services, even in a 'free at the time of use' service such as the British NHS, tend to be provided in inverse proportion to the needs of the local population – the so-called 'inverse care law'.[54] The evidence was based on the better access to better health services enjoyed by the more privileged sections of the UK population, with more highly qualified and innovative practitioners and better facilities in more affluent areas compared with more pathology and medical need in more deprived areas.

In the USA, where payment is required and lack of insurance leads to exclusion from healthcare, the operation of the inverse care law is obvious. Those with adequate insurance and/or sufficient financial resources have access to 'state of the art' medical treatment, whilst many of the poor and native Americans are dependent on special government-funded insurance programmes to cover medical expenses.[55] I   '% (9 million) of US children had no insurance, ⟨   ⟩ or public (Medicaid).[55] Over 20% of children wh   ⟩r poor or near-poor were uninsured and not c⟨   ⟩Medicaid.[55] Hispanic children were the ethnic group ⟨   ⟩st percentage of uninsured children. Among adult⟨   ⟩limitation due to chronic conditions, 16.6% we   in 1989 although only 1% of those with severe d⟨   ⟩o cover.[55]

In less developed countries, those mos⟨   ⟩ealthcare are least likely to have access to it. This ap⟨   ⟩rly to the rural poor, who often have no health s⟨   ⟩he urban poor may also be excluded from the expe⟨   ⟩ palaces' which have been built in many major c⟨   ⟩eveloped countries.[56] Based on the United Natio⟨   ⟩ent Programme's definition of health service access (the percentage of the population able to reach appropriate local health services on foot or by local means of transport in no more than one hour), more than one-third of the population of less developed countries had no access to health services at the end of the 1980s and this percentage rose to almost 50% for the countries of sub-Saharan Africa.[57]

The Declaration of Alma Ata was devoted to the provision of primary healthcare to all communities in ways which ensured comprehensive access to services relevant to the needs of the community.[58] However, a number of factors have conspired to frustrate the realisation of the WHO's plan for comprehensive primary care: less developed countries have limited resources to spend on health and many spend very small proportions of their per capita GNP on health; even in those countries striving to provide primary healthcare services to their populations, these efforts have been frustrated in recent years by the policies of the international funding agencies (IMF and the World Bank), which have promoted privatisation of health facilities, greater reliance on health insurance, more use of direct charges to patients and service users and administrative decentralisation of healthcare.[14,57,59]

Thus, there is evidence that the poor, whose need for health services is often greater, are less likely to have access to them in both developed and less developed countries of the world. This is despite the fact that primary child healthcare services, especially in less developed countries, are known to improve health and life expectancy and are relatively cheap to deliver.[60] As considered in Chapter 5, those poorer countries which have achieved low infant and child mortality rates and life expectancy equivalent to those of developed countries have done so, in part, by prioritising primary healthcare for mothers and children.[38]

In developed countries such as the UK, where health service access is not limited by ability to pay, there are other more subtle barriers to their use by the poor. Access to many services is by telephone and many families in deprived areas lack a telephone.[61] Lack of transport and the problem of organising substitute care for dependants also present barriers to healthcare use for the poor.[61] Even when these barriers are overcome, there are others to surmount. Doctors in primary and secondary care are frequently 'protected' by receptionists who 'filter' enquiries. Class and language barriers can also impede health service access.

Despite the barriers considered above, poor families tend to make greater use of illness services for their children, with higher primary care consultation rates and rates of hospital admission.[34,62] However, these same families make less use of preventive services, including dental, health surveillance and immunisation services.[34] They are labelled 'non-attenders' and are often seen as 'inconsiderate' as they divert scarce health service resources from others who could have used them.[63] When reasons for low uptake of preventive services are more closely studied, they show that families with limited resources, rather than lacking consideration or knowledge, frequently make rational choices related to available financial and time resources.[61,64]

The role of other social divisions in exacerbating the effects of poverty on health

Racism as an exacerbating factor and a mediating mechanism between poverty and ill health has been considered in Chapter 7. Minority families and their children tend to suffer the double jeopardy of the health effects of poverty and the stress and psychosocial affront associated with racism. At the same income levels, minority families are more likely to live in poor overcrowded housing conditions and experience more difficulty accessing health and social care facilities.[65] Employment opportunities are more restricted and even those with high qualifications experience racism in gaining access to the professions or obtaining posts once they are qualified within those professions.[66] Insult is added to injury when black Americans are informed by some researchers that they are genetically inferior in intelligence and are contributing to the development of an 'underclass' which is held responsible for all the social ills of present-day America (also *see* Chapter 6).[67]

Gender continues to act as a factor which deepens and exacerbates the experience of poverty in both developed and less developed countries. Women, even in countries where female emancipation has apparently been established for a number of generations, continue to carry the main burden of caring within the family and often sacrifice their own health and well-being to protect their children from the worst effects of poverty and social exclusion.[11] They may experience 'hidden' poverty as a result of maldistribution of available resources within the home (*see* Chapter 1, p. 5) and, in some societies, female children and women are discriminated against in the distribution of limited food.[68,69]

Women, because of their main caring role, tend to be held responsible for health problems which affect their children. The earlier research emphasis on maternal incompetence/ inefficiency represented one extreme of this victim-blaming approach, but the same underlying message of inadequacy of individual care and individual blame are implicit in the health education messages which focus on maternal smoking without acknowledging the social context in which smoking takes place. Similarly, the exhortations of former UK government ministers to poor mothers to 'shop around and buy cheaper foods' are not merely insulting but serve to further exclude these families from the mainstream.[70]

Young single mothers have been attacked by politicians in the UK and USA and accused of planning pregnancy in order to gain welfare advantages.[71] In the UK, their actions are seen as the main driving force in the development of the so-called 'underclass'; they join black Americans in sharing the blame in the USA.[72] There is no evidence to support the contentions and assumptions underlying these assertions (*see* Chapter 6, p. 158); in fact, what evidence there is suggests that lack of job opportunities plays a significant part in pushing young women towards child bearing as a 'career'.[73,74] Victim-blaming of this nature serves only to further undermine self-esteem and increase social isolation.

Another group who have suffered exclusion and social isolation are the disabled. With some notable exceptions, such as Sweden, disability reduces chances of employment and pushes many individuals and families into poverty. The psychosocial effects of disability itself can be considerable, but these are frequently accentuated by social exclusion and stigma.

Cumulative effects of lifetime social circumstances and inter-generational influences

The foregoing discussion illustrates some of the possible mechanisms by which poverty and low SES may adversely affect health. None of these factors alone can account for the burden of ill health attributable to social inequalities, nor can they account for the fine grading of the association of SES with many child health outcomes in developed (Chapter 6) and less developed (Chapter 5) countries. If, however, the cumulative effects of these factors at any one time and over the individual's lifetime are considered then it begins to be possible to explain both the extent and the patterning of health inequalities.[1,22] In the case of children and, to a lesser extent, adults, inter-generational effects need to be added to social factors acting within the child's own lifetime.

Cross-sectionally, advantage and disadvantage in one aspect of life is likely to be accompanied by similar advantage or disadvantage in other aspects.[75] Data from the 1958 UK National Cohort Study illustrate this effect. Mean height attained at 11 years was 13 cm less in children from multiply disadvantaged families with a range of adverse social factors than children with none of these disadvantages.[76] Children with some but fewer disadvantages had mean heights which were distributed between the extremes. Data from the National Longitudinal Survey of Youth and the Infant Health and Development Program in the USA show that children in families with incomes less than half of the poverty threshold scored 6–13 points lower on various standardised tests of IQ, verbal activity and achievement than those living in families with incomes between 1.5 and twice the poverty threshold.[77] A dose–response relationship was noted with different income levels. Families with incomes less than half the poverty threshold are known to suffer multiple disadvantage.

Advantages and disadvantages accumulate over time in a simple additive fashion and, in some cases, the factors are synergistic, leading to a multiplier effect.[1] Figure 9.1 shows the cumulative effects over time of disadvantage on educational

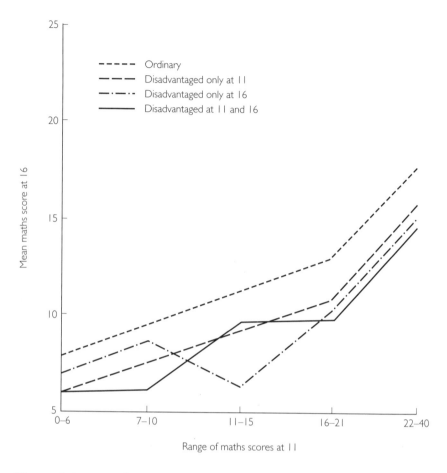

Figure 9.1   Disadvantage and mean maths scores at age 16 for a given range of maths scores at 11.

attainment in children from the 1958 UK National Cohort.[76] Children disadvantaged at 11 and 16 years had the lowest educational attainment at both ages and showed no tendency to catch up between the two ages. The effect of long-term poverty on children's cognitive ability has been shown to be greater than that associated with short-term poverty and living above the poverty threshold.[78] Many studies have identified the effects of childhood socio-economic position on health in adult life.[79–81] Lynch *et al.*[82] report results from the Kuopio Ischaemic Heart Disease Risk Factor Study in Finland which show that many adult behaviours, such as smoking, and psychosocial dispositions detrimental to health are consistently related to poor childhood conditions and low levels of education. These studies support the contention that risks and protective factors cluster over the life course.

Life course research has focused mainly on the effects of social childhood conditions on adult health.[83] However, health in infancy and childhood is strongly influenced by the parental, particularly the maternal, cumulated life course experience. The social gradient in birth weight[84,85] is the result of the fine grading of advantages and disadvantages originating as far back as the mother's own experience as a fetus, through her own childhood and into pregnancy.[86,87] Interventions designed to improve pregnancy outcomes are unlikely to meet with success if they focus on one risk factor, such as smoking or diet, without taking account of the cumulative effects of the mother's life course. A woman whose parents were disadvantaged is more likely to have been low birth weight herself; to have experienced more childhood ill health; to have had a less nutritious diet with adverse effects on her growth leading to relative stunting and anaemia; to have started smoking in adolescence and be less likely to quit in early pregnancy; and to come to pregnancy at an earlier age. The more disadvantaged the woman the more likely she is to have experienced increasing numbers of risk factors and fewer protective factors. It is scientifically unsatisfactory and implausible to attribute the low birth weight of a mother such as this to smoking alone. As acknowledged by the Acheson Report,[88] interventions aimed at improving neonatal health need to start in the mother's childhood.

These cumulative influences of disadvantage have been conceptualised in terms of theories of 'general susceptibility/vulnerability' to disease in low socio-economic groups, mediated through many of the determinants considered above and having a final common pathway in physiological mechanisms which suppress the immune system.[89–91] General susceptibility would seem to explain many of the differences in health outcomes associated with disadvantage. Blaxter concludes from her study of health and lifestyles that 'a general susceptibility, clearly linked to socio-economic situation, is being demonstrated' (p. 240).[92] Hart, in a re-analysis of the data related to the Dutch Hunger

Winter of 1944–45, demonstrates that the relative advantage of community over a long period of time can provide protection against acute adversity, concluding that:

> The children of the Dutch Hunger Winter who survived to record the highest vitality and durability in the post-war Netherlands were born in the worst-affected part of the country, but surely to mothers whose material circumstances during growth and development in childhood had been relatively privileged. Moreover, they were the latest descendants of one of Europe's oldest and most sophisticated urban populations. ([28] p. 45)

Smith and co-workers caution that general susceptibility is not supported by the wide heterogeneity of strength and direction of association in the socio-economic distribution of cancers in particular sites, and argue that:

> Attempts to account for social class differences in health might be usefully conceptualised in terms of the balance between general susceptibility and specific aetiology, with consideration given to which part of the relationship is being influenced by any explanatory variable. ([22] p. 141)

From the above, it is evident that the search for single causative agents in the explanation of health inequalities is doomed to failure and the techniques of analysis used are likely to create the false impression that one variable is 'independently' associated with an outcome or 'accounts for' the effect of another.[93] Causal models and pathways which reflect the complexity of the relation between multiple factors acting at different times are a more fruitful way of conceptualising the process by which health inequalities arise and are perpetuated.

Causal models and pathways

Most causal models assume that variables can be classified according to the level at which their influence seems to be exerted:

variables which act at some distance from the outcome of interest are referred to as *distal* and typically include economic, political and socio-cultural factors beyond the immediate control of the family; other variables which mediate between the macro-environment and the immediate environment of the child are referred to as *intermediate* and typically include child care practices, food distribution within the household and exposure to pathogens; those variables which are directly responsible for disease, such as specific pathogens and smoking, are classified as *proximal*. Rose uses a simpler concept of *proximal* and *underlying* causes or *causes of causes*.[94] Whatever the terminology and the number of levels identified, the basic concept acknowledges that causal disease agents do not act alone and are part of a complex web of factors functioning at different levels.

Millard uses three levels to model the causes of high rates of child mortality, with particular reference to less developed countries. Her model concentrates on international and national economic factors at the distal level influencing household food, security and water supply (ultimate tier), which in turn influences food distribution within the family and children's diets (intermediate tier), finally leading into the cycle of malnutrition, respiratory infection, diarrhoea and ultimately death (Figure 9.2).[95]

Waxler and co-workers, in attempting to explain infant mortality in Sri Lankan households, state:

> *In each set of variables that we have examined, medical, social and ethnic, we have found several that are significant predictors of infant deaths in the sampled Sri Lankan families. For example, lack of sanitary latrine is associated with infant mortality; poverty and poor education are associated with infant mortality; minority group status is associated with infant mortality. Each of these predictors of infant death is empirically linked with the others as well. Lack of sanitary latrines are most common among poor and uneducated families; poverty and lack of education are characteristic of minority cultural groups. To understand how these variables work together and to*

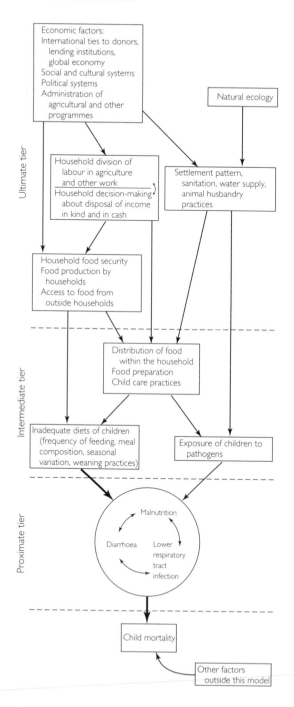

Figure 9.2   Three-tier causal model of child mortality.
(Source [95] p. 255)

determine which ones have the greatest predictive weight, we have constructed a path model that looks concurrently at the ethnic, economic, educational and medical explanations of infant deaths. ([96] p. 389)

Their path model is shown in Figure 9.3. However, this is only able to explain 5% of the variance and the authors acknowledge that this would be expected because they are using individual rather than aggregated data and they have been highly selective in their choice of variables. However, they are able to demonstrate a series of causally related links which best explain infant deaths in the sample of families studied, which they summarise as 'Minority group status results in poverty, which prevents people from having safe sanitary facilities, which causes infant deaths'.

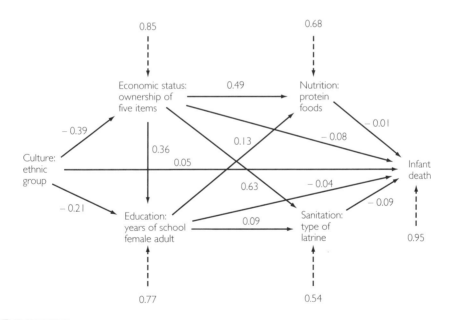

Figure 9.3   Path model showing cultural, socio-economic and medical predictors of infant death in 480 Sri Lankan households. All the figures refer to correlation coefficients (direct effects only). The figures on the periphery with dotted line arrows represent the amount of variance *unexplained* by the variables in the model. (Source [96] p. 389)

Path analysis has been used to study the relationship between socio-economic status and infant mortality in the USA.[97,98] Using this methodology, Brooks[97] was able to demonstrate that socio-economic factors determine variations in country infant mortality, neonatal mortality and post-neonatal mortality rates and to challenge suggestions that socio-economic correlations with infant mortality were in decline. Sheehan uses a structural modelling approach to study the relationship between stress and low birth weight.[99] Figure 9.4a and b shows the structural equation model of stress factors affecting low birth weight and the best model of the influence of stress on birth weight, which suggests that economic stress is mediated through lack of social support and family stress which in turn act through addictive behaviour (smoking and drinking alcohol) to affect birth weight. As Sheehan states, 'structural equation modelling can provide insight into a complex set of relationships by examining combinations of remote and proximal relationships' (p. 1510). However, causal pathways should be treated with caution as they suffer the same problems of causal attribution as other analyses based on empirical observation. Their advantage lies in their capacity to conceptualise and study complex relationships between distal and proximal predictor variables.

A theoretical framework for the analysis of causal relationships in child health

From the above discussion of causal mechanisms, it is possible to begin to draw up a theoretical framework for analysing causal relationships in child health. The framework must take into account a range of variables which interact over time and may have a cause–effect relationship (in other words may be 'causes of causes'). It must incorporate a number of levels reflecting distal as well as proximal influences on health outcomes. It should set health outcomes within a causal pathway which accounts not only for the most proximal influences but considers distal factors at an international and national level which, mediated through other variables, might influence how

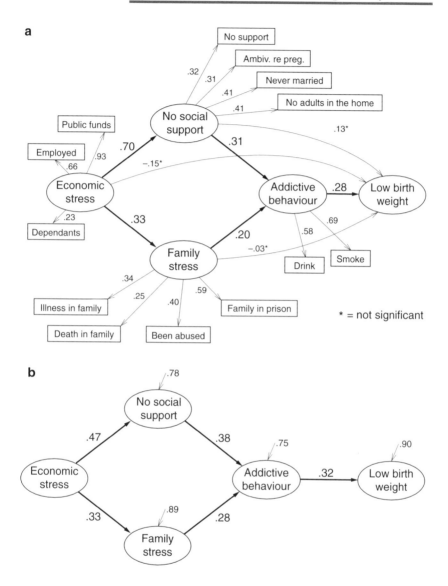

Figure 9.4   (a) Structural equation model of stress factors affecting low birth weight; (b) best model of influence of stress factors on low birth weight. (Source [99] pp. 1508–9)

families function at a micro level. To take an extreme example, the nutritional choices open to families in the Dutch Hunger Winter were influenced directly by internationally taken decisions totally beyond their individual control. For many families in less developed countries, decisions taken by the World Bank and the IMF directly influence local food prices and access to education and healthcare. Though usually more subtle, the influence exerted by international economic movements may have a direct effect on household consumption in developed countries as well – for example, the catastrophic world slump in the 1930s directly affected millions of households throughout the developed world, causing hardship and poverty due to unemployment, and though the effects of the recent world recession have been less dramatic, these economic changes at an international level have exerted profound effects on families, particularly those in the traditional centres of heavy industry in Europe and the USA.

Thus, a theoretical framework which addresses complex causal processes must move away from the dominant idea of a single causal agent working in isolation at a short distance physically and in time from the outcome. The 'single cause' approach appeared to be remarkably successful in relation to some of the infectious diseases which were prominent in developed countries in the 19th century but, as considered in Chapter 4, the medical treatments flowing from the single cause theory had less effect on mortality and morbidity than social and public health changes, and has always been inadequate in explaining why some people become ill as a result of infection and others do not.[100] Causal pathways allow mediators to be set in a social and environmental context as well as accounting for changes induced by international and national health and social policies. Part of their importance is that they set potential solutions within the same international and national political and social context. Health and social policies influencing poverty and child health are the subject of the next part of the book.

Summary

1   There are historically and scientifically plausible mechanisms by which poverty and low SES may influence health outcomes, including unemployment, underemployment,

poor housing, debt, suboptimal nutrition and a range of psychological factors such as powerlessness, self-esteem and financially-induced alienation from consumerism.

2   These mechanisms are unlikely to exert their influence on health discretely. Many of the poor in developed and less developed countries experience multiple disadvantage and deprivation, and the effects of these factors are likely to be cumulative and act across as well as within generations.

3   Single causal factors are unable to account for these cumulative effects and are therefore limited in their ability to explain causal mechanisms in the relation between health and SES.

4   Causal pathways and models which accommodate the cumulative influence of various factors over time are more likely to offer a fruitful approach to explaining the relation between health and SES.

References

1   Shaw M, Dorling D, Gordon D *et al.* (1999) *The Widening Gap: Health Inequalities and Policy in Britain.* The Policy Press, University of Bristol, Bristol.

2   Smith GD and Morris JK (1994) Increasing inequalities in the health of the nation. *BMJ.* **309**:1453–4.

3   Sloggett A and Joshi H (1994) Higher mortality in deprived areas: community or personal disadvantage. *BMJ.* **309**:1470–4.

4   Townsend P (1994) The rich man in his castle. *BMJ.* **309**: 1674–5.

5   Duncan GJ, Brooks-Gunn J and Klebanov PK (1994) Economic deprivation and early childhood development. *Child Dev.* **65**:296–318.

6   Baum A, Fleming R and Reddy DM (1986) Unemployment stress: loss of control, reactance and learned helplessness. *Soc. Sci. Med.* 5:509–16.

7   Berthoud R and Kempson E (1990) *Credit and Debt: First Findings of the PSI Survey.* Policy Studies Institute, London.

8   Graham H (1994) Breadline motherhood: trends and experiences in Ireland. *Administration.* 42(4):352–73.

9   National Consumer Council (NCC) (1990) *Credit and Debt: The Consumer Interest.* HMSO, London.

10   National Children's Homes (1992) *Deep in Debt: A Survey of Problems Faced by Low Income Families.* NCH, London.

11   Graham H (1993) Smoking among working class women. *Primary Health Care.* 3(2):15–16.

12   Research Unit in Health and Behavioural Change (RUHBC) (1989) *Changing the Public Health.* Wiley, Chichester.

13   Ineichen B (1993) *Homes and Health: How Housing and Health Interact.* EFN Spon, London.

14   Godlee F (1993) Third world debt. *BMJ.* 307:1369–70.

15   Heath I (1994) The poor man at his gate. *BMJ.* 309:1675–6.

16   Gray A (ed.) (1993) *World Health and Disease.* Open University Press, Milton Keynes.

17   Department of Social Policy, University of Newcastle (1991) *The Walker Riverside Study: Report and Recommendations.* Newcastle University, Newcastle upon Tyne.

18   Chamberlin R (ed.) (1988) *Beyond Individual Risk Assessment: Community-wide Approaches to Promoting the Health and Development of Families and Children.* The National Center for Education in Maternal and Child Health, Washington DC.

19 Graydon R (1989) High-risk children. *Child Safety Review* [Newsletter of the Child Accident Prevention Trust]. **1/Summer**: 3.

20 Oakley A, Rigby AS and Hickey D (1993) Women and children last? Class, health and the role of maternal and child health services. *Eur. J. Public Health.* **3**:220–6.

21 Brown GW and Harris T (1978) *Social Origins of Depression: A Study of Psychiatric Disorder in Women.* Tavistock, London.

22 Smith GD, Blane D and Bartley M (1994) Explanations of socio-economic differences in mortality: evidence from Britain and elsewhere. *Eur. J. Public Health.* **4**:131–44.

23 Kleinman RE, Murphy JM, Little M *et al.* (1998) Hunger in children in the United States: potential behavioral and emotional correlates. *Pediatrics.* **101**:E3.

24 Wynn A and Wynn M (1981) *The Prevention of Handicap of Early Pregnancy Origin.* Foundation for Education and Research in Child-rearing, London.

25 Baird D (1974) The epidemiology of low birth weight: changes in incidence in Aberdeen 1948–72. *J. Biosoc. Sci.* **7**:77–97.

26 Aukett MA and Wharton BA (1995) Suboptimal nutrition. In *Social Paediatrics* (eds B Lindstrom and NJ Spencer). Oxford University Press, Oxford.

27 Nelson M (1999) Nutrition and health inequalities. In *Inequalities in Health* (eds D Gordon, M Shaw, D Dorling *et al.*). The Policy Press, University of Bristol, Bristol.

28 Hart N (1993) Famine, maternal nutrition and infant mortality: a re-examination of the Dutch Hunger Winter. *Popul. Stud.* **47**:27–46.

29 Hoffman HJ, Damus K, Hillman L *et al.* (1988) Risk factors for SIDS: results in the National Institute of Child Health

and Human Development SIDS cooperative epidemiological study. In *The Sudden Infant Death Syndrome: Cardiac and Respiratory Mechanisms and Interventions* (eds PJ Schwartz, DP Southall and M Valdez-Dapena). *Ann. NY Acad. Sci.* 533:13–30.

30 Caldwell J and McDonald P (1982) Influence of maternal education in infant and child mortality: levels and causes. *Popul. Stud.* 33:395–413.

31 Palloni A (1981) Mortality in Latin America: emerging patterns. *Popul. Dev. Rev.* 7(4):623–49.

32 Garrett P, Ng'andu N and Ferron J (1994) Poverty experiences of young children and the quality of their home environments. *Child Develop.* 65:331–45.

33 Sampson RJ and Laub JH (1994) Urban poverty and the family context of delinquency: a new look at structures and process in a classic study. *Child Develop.* 65:523–40.

34 Jolly DL (1990) *The Impact of Adversity on Child Health – Poverty and Disadvantage*. Australian College of Paediatrics, Parkville, Victoria.

35 Rutter M and Smith D (eds) (1995) *Psychosocial Disorders in Young People*. Wiley, Chichester.

36 Aukett MA, Parks YA, Scott PH *et al.* (1986) Treatment with iron increases weight gain and psychomotor development. *Arch. Dis. Child.* 61:849–57.

37 Spencer NJ (1984) Parents' identification of the ill child. In *Progress in Child Health* (ed. JA McFarlane). Churchill Livingstone, Edinburgh.

38 United Nations Development Programme (1994) *Human Development Report*. UNDP and Oxford University Press, New York.

39 Costello A, Watson F and Woodward D (1994) *Human Faces or Human Facade? Adjustment and the Health of Mothers*

and Children. Centre for International Child Health, Institute of Child Health, London.

40 Wilkinson RG (1996) *Unhealthy Societies. The Afflictions of Inequality.* Routledge, London.

41 Marmot M and Wilkinson RG (eds) (1999*) Social Determinants of Health*. Oxford University Press, Oxford.

42 Martin C, Platt SD and Hunt SM (1987) Housing and ill health. *BMJ.* **294**:1125–7.

43 Wilkinson RG (1991) *The Impact of Inequality on Health*. Paper presented at annual conference of British Sociological Association.

44 Huston AC, McLoyd VC and Cull CG (1994) Children and poverty: issues in contemporary research. *Child Develop.* **65**:275–82.

45 Berkman LF and Syme SL (1979) Social network, host resistance and mortality: a nine-year follow up study of Alameda County residents. *Am. J. Epidemiol.* **109**:186–204.

46 Hoghugi M and Speight ANP (1998) Good enough parenting for all children – a strategy for a healthier society. *Arch. Dis. Child.* **78**:293–6.

47 Thwaites EJ and Sutherland I (1951) A method of assessing maternal efficiency for socio-medical surveys. *Arch. Dis. Child.* **27**:60–6.

48 Burns BL (1947) Home and social environmental factors and the health of the school child. *J. Roy. Inst. Public Health.* **10**:325–36.

49 Miller FJW, Court SDM, Knox EG *et al.* (1974) *The School Years in Newcastle upon Tyne*. Oxford University Press, Oxford.

50 Taylor J, Spencer NJ and Baldwin N (2000) The social, economic and political context of parenting. *Arch. Dis. Child.* **82**:113–20.

51 Stansfeld SA (1999) Social support and social cohesion. In *Social Determinants of Health* (eds M Marmot and RG Wilkinson). Oxford University Press, Oxford.

52 Kawachi I and Kennedy BP (1997) Income distribution, social capital and mortality. In *Socioeconomic Inequalities and Health* (eds P Crampton and P Howden-Chapman). Institute of Policy Studies, Victoria University of Wellington, New Zealand.

53 Tung-liang C (1999) Economic transition and changing relation between income inequality and mortality in Taiwan: regression analysis. *BMJ*. **319**:1162–5.

54 Tudor Hart J (1971) The inverse care law. *Lancet*. **27 Feb**: 405–12.

55 Lillie-Blanton M, Martinez RM, Lyons B *et al.* (1999) *Access to Health Care: Promises and Prospects for Low-income Americans*. The Kaiser Commission on Medicaid and the Uninsured, Washington DC.

56 Ebrahim GJ (1985) *Social and Community Paediatrics in Developing Countries*. Macmillan, London.

57 Webster C (ed.) (1993) *Caring for Health: History and Diversity*. Open University Press, Milton Keynes.

58 World Health Organization (1978) *Reports of the International Conference on Primary Health Care, Alma Ata, USSR, 6–12 September*. WHO, Geneva.

59 Logie DE and Woodroffe J (1993) Structural adjustment: the wrong prescription for Africa? *BMJ*. **307**:41–4.

60 World Health Organization (1995) *The World Health Report*. WHO, Geneva.

61 Pearson M, Dawson C, Moore H *et al.* (1992) Health on borrowed time? Prioritizing and meeting needs in low-income households. *Health Soc. Care*. **1**:45–54.

62   Spencer NJ, Logan S, Scholey S *et al.* (1996) Deprivation and bronchiolitis. *Arch. Dis. Child.* 74:50–2.

63   Darling WM (1991) Chairman's speech given to the Annual Conference of the National Association of Health Authorities and Trusts, 26 June 1991, Bournemouth, England.

64   Mayall B and Foster MC (1989) *Child Health Care: Living with Children; Working for Children.* Heinemann Nursing, Oxford.

65   Smaje C (1995) *Health, Race and Ethnicity: Making Sense of the Evidence.* King's Fund Institute, London.

66   Esmail A and Etherington S (1993) Racial discrimination against doctors from ethnic minorities. *BMJ.* 306:691–2.

67   Murray C and Herrnstein R (1994) *The Bell Curve: Intelligence and Class Structure in American Life.* The Free Press, New York.

68   Engle P L (1993) Influences of mother's and father's income on children's nutritional status in Guatemala. *Soc. Sci. Med.* 37:1303–12.

69   Babu SC, Thirumaran S and Mohanam TC (1993) Agricultural productivity, seasonality and gender bias in rural nutrition: empirical evidence from South India. *Soc. Sci. Med.* 37:1313–19.

70   Widdecombe A (1991) Comments in response to NCH Poverty and Nutrition Survey. *The Guardian,* 4th June, 1991.

71   Leach P (1994) *Children First.* Michael Joseph, London.

72   Green P (1981) *The Pursuit of Inequality.* Pantheon Books, New York.

73   Spencer NJ (1994) Teenage mothers. *Curr. Paediatr.* 4:48–51.

74   Penhale B (1989) *Associations between unemployment and fertility among young women in the early 1980s*. Longitudinal study working paper No. 60. OPCS, London.

75   Blane D (1999) The life course, the social gradient and health. In *Social Determinants of Health* (eds M Marmot and RG Wilkinson). Oxford University Press, Oxford.

76   Davie R, Butler N and Goldstein H (1972) *From Birth to Seven*. Longmans, London.

77   Smith JR, Brooks-Gunn J and Klebanov P (1997) The consequences of living in poverty for young children's cognitive and verbal ability and early schooling achievement. In *Consequences of Growing Up Poor* (eds GJ Duncan and J Brooks-Gunn). Russell Sage Foundation, New York.

78   Korenman S, Miller JE and Sjaastad JE (1995) Long-term poverty and child development in the United States: results from the National Longitudinal Survey of Youth. *Child. Youth Serv. Rev.* 17:127–51.

79   Forsdahl A (1977) Are poor living conditions in childhood and adolescence an important risk factor for arteriosclerotic heart disease? *Br. J. Prevent. Soc. Med.* 31:91–5.

80   Kaplan GA and Salonen JT (1990) Socioeconomic conditions in childhood and ischaemic heart disease during middle age. *BMJ.* 301:1121–3.

81   Nystrom Peck M (1994) The importance of childhood socioeconomic group for adult health. *Soc. Sci. Med.* 39:553–62.

82   Lynch JW, Kaplan GW and Salonen JT (1997) Why do poor people behave poorly? Variation in adult health behaviors and psychosocial characteristics by stages of the socioeconomic lifecourse. *Soc. Sci. Med.* 44:809–19.

83   Kuh D and Ben-Shlomo Y (1997) *A life-course approach to chronic disease epidemiology*. Oxford University Press, Oxford.

84 Spencer NJ, Bambang S, Logan S *et al.* (1999) Socio-economic status and birth weight: comparison of an area-based measure with the Registrar General's social class. *J. Epidemiol. Community Health.* **53**:495–8.

85 Elmen H, Hoglund D, Karlberg P *et al.* (1996) Birth weight for gestational age as a health indicator: birth weight and mortality measures at the local area level. *Eur. J. Public Health.* **6**:137–41.

86 Hackman E, Emanuel I, van Belle G *et al.* (1983) Maternal birth weight and subsequent pregnancy outcome. *JAMA.* **250**:2016–19.

87 Baird D (1980) Environment and reproduction. *Br. J. Obstet. Gynaecol.* **87**:1057–67.

88 Department of Health (1998) *Independent Inquiry into Inequalities in Health (the Acheson Report).* The Stationery Office, London.

89 Susser MW, Watson W and Hopper K (1985) *Sociology in Medicine.* Oxford University Press, New York.

90 Najman JM (1980) Theories of disease causation and the concept of a general susceptibility: a review. *Soc. Sci. Med.* **14A**:231–7.

91 Jemmott JB and Locke SE (1984) Psychosocial factors, immunologic mediation and human susceptibility to infectious diseases: how much do we know? *Psychol. Bull.* **95**:78–108.

92 Blaxter M (1990) *Health and Lifestyles.* Tavistock/Routledge, London and New York.

93 Smith GD and Phillips AN (1992) Confounding in epidemiological studies: why 'independent' effects may not be all they seem. *BMJ.* **305**:757–9.

94 Rose G (1992) *The Strategy of Preventive Medicine.* Oxford University Press, Oxford.

95 Millard AV (1994) A causal model of high rates of child mortality. *Soc. Sci. Med.* **38**:253–68.

96 Waxler NE, Morrison BM, Sirisena WM *et al.* (1985) Infant mortality in Sri Lankan households: a causal model. *Soc. Sci. Med.* **20**:381–92.

97 Brooks CH (1975) Path analysis of socioeconomic correlates of country infant mortality rates. *Int. J. Health Serv.* **5**:499–514.

98 Brooks CH (1980) Social, economic and biologic correlates of infant mortality in city neighborhoods. *J. Health Soc. Behav.* **21**:2–11.

99 Sheehan TJ (1998) Stress and low birth weight: a structural modeling approach using real life stressors. *Soc. Sci. Med.* **47**:1503–12.

100 Najman JM (1980) Theories of disease causation and the concept of a general susceptibility: a review. *Soc. Sci. Med.* **14A**:231–7.

Part Four

Social and health policy implications

10

Social policy implications

Introduction

If structural explanations for health inequalities best fit the historical and global evidence, as argued in the previous section, it follows that political solutions based on health and social policy are likely to be more effective than health education and medical and pharmacological interventions, however well organised. This is not to argue that medically based interventions are of no value, but realisation of their potential benefits is dependent on the political and economic climate in which they are being practised.[1-3] Thus, there are national and international health and social policy implications in tackling the effects of poverty on child health.

This chapter will address these implications first by a historical review of British social and health policy provision for poverty and its health consequences. Second, social policies and their negative and positive effects on health inequalities will be discussed. Finally, the features of national and international social policies which are necessary to combat the adverse health effects of poverty and low socio-economic status (SES) will be summarised. The following chapter looks at specific health service interventions and future research priorities.

Historical review of social policy and its relation to health

The Elizabethan or Old Poor Law

As a result of epidemics and economic decline as many as 20% of the population in 16th-century English towns could be identified as poor.[4] National legislation was eventually enacted in 1598 and 1601, now known as the Old Poor Law, which provided welfare and some healthcare for the poor. Each parish (local council) was responsible for its own poor, who were to be supported by a compulsory poor rate which was set by and levied upon the parish's most prosperous householders.[4] An important distinction was made in this legislation between 'able-bodied' poor and the 'impotent' poor, those such as children, the elderly and the disabled, who were unable to look after themselves. Because of their inability to care for themselves, the impotent poor were entitled to poor relief as of right from the parish in which they were born.[5] The able-bodied poor, on the other hand, could only receive relief by undertaking supervised work in the Houses of Correction, the underlying philosophy of which was that their inability to provide for themselves and their families reflected an inadequate work motivation and this attitude was in need of 'correction'.[5]

The New Poor Law

The rapid industrialisation which occurred in the late 18th century led to an upsurge in the numbers in poverty.[5] This, combined with the increasing need to supplement the wages of those in employment (so-called 'outdoor' relief) and the transformation of many of the Houses of Correction into places of detention for the insane, the aged and the infirm, forced a reappraisal of the whole system.[5] A Royal Commission, established in 1832 and including liberal reformers such as Edwin Chadwick, was responsible for formulating the New Poor Law, designed to overcome the perceived shortcomings of the Elizabethan Law.

The New Poor Law of 1834 was aimed particularly at the able-bodied poor and reflected the individualistic beliefs and values of the rising class of manufacturers and professionals that each person was responsible for their own actions and their own well-being.[5] The Law stressed deterrence rather than entitlement and sought to overcome the crisis created by the burgeoning need for outdoor relief created by low wages by reasserting institutional measures for dealing with the able-bodied poor.[4] To eliminate outdoor relief in the form of supplementation of depressed wages in the agricultural south of England, a so-called 'workhouse test' was instituted under which the poor, in order to obtain relief, had to be desperate enough to enter the workhouse, which had to be 'less eligible' (more distasteful) than any work available outside the workhouse.[4] Workhouses, larger than the Houses of Correction they replaced, were created by Poor Law Unions, amalgamations of a number of parishes, with a central administration.

The New Law stigmatised the poor by obliging them to wear uniforms, separating wives from husbands and children from parents, and subjecting them to strict and monotonous regimes.[5] The poor lost their personal freedom and, when the franchise was extended in 1867 and 1884, were excluded from the vote.[5] Despite these draconian measures to eliminate outdoor relief, local discretion ensured that the able-bodied poor were often given outdoor relief which was cheaper, and the workhouses, like the Houses of Correction before them, became full of those seen as being incapable of helping themselves and those who became known as the 'undeserving' poor, such as mothers of illegitimate children or vagrants. The elderly and infirm sections of the 'deserving' poor were offered sick relief in Poor Law Infirmaries.

Sanitarianism and the Public Health Movement

Alongside the enforcement of the New Poor Law, the sanitary movement developed. The newly instituted Poor Law Unions, in addition to their responsibilities administering the workhouses, were expected to undertake sanitary improvements and vaccination.[4] Sanitary improvements were aimed at cleansing, watering, sewering and rehousing populations, especially in large towns. Pressure for these improvements arose from increased understanding of the role of insanitary conditions in epidemics such as cholera as well as the realisation from the work of Chadwick and others that the poor were more vulnerable to death and illness.[4] Like the New Poor Law, part of the aim of the movement was to reduce wasteful expenditure as well as prevent the diseases which reduced the earning capacity of the labouring classes.

The sanitary movement contributed to the development of the Public Health Movement, which led to the appointment of Medical Officers of Health and national legislation culminating in the Public Health Act of 1848. Despite the momentum established by the sanitary movement, its passage was not entirely trouble free: the national General Board of Health, established by the 1848 Act, was short-lived owing to opposition from strong vested interests to centralised health administration.[4]

An important element of the public health legislation was the regulation of building, with national standards of house construction. However, much of this legislation was ignored until the Housing, Town Planning Act of 1909.[6] Measures to ensure maintenance of property (the Torrens Act 1868) and to encourage slum clearance (the Cross Act 1875) led to slow improvement in housing conditions.[6] However, overcrowding, perhaps the single most important determinant of the spread of infectious illness, was difficult to eradicate; for example, in Scotland 64% of the population in 1861 lived in one- or two-roomed houses.[6]

Public health and housing legislation did not benefit those in greatest need for some time, primarily because it was initially voluntary, was opposed by powerful financial and local interests and, even when mandatory, poorly enforced. For example, 'back-to-back' housing, restricted in local bye-laws in the mid-19th century and outlawed in the 1909 Town Planning Act, continued to be built by the local administration in Leeds until 1937.[6]

Child labour contributed significantly to ill health and early death in the newly industrialised British towns. Factory inspectors were introduced, and under legislation introduced in

1833 it became illegal to employ children below the age of nine in factories.

With the discovery that cholera was water-borne, water and sewage became preoccupations of the Public Health Movement. Here, as with housing, sanitary improvements met with resistance from local vested interests, as shown by this quote from the Rev. Dare of Leicester in 1852:

> *The completion of the Water Works will be a great blessing to the town …. From the far villas on the London-road, to the extremities of 'the North' and the Belgrave-gate, fever and diarrhoea have spread their desolate blight. From these and other causes vast numbers of the poor are always in a low state of health. This is no doubt the reason why they are perpetually seeking after the nostrums of quackery. Of course, I have heard of the 'Wise Woman of Wing'. The London Board, by its dilatoriness and needless objections to the proposed Drainage Scheme, has been the best patron she has had in this neighbourhood.* ([7] pp. 43–4)

The private water companies resisted legislation aimed at forcing them to draw water from sources free from contamination by sewage and, of interest in the light of recent water privatisation in the UK, municipalisation of water companies was seen as a triumph of public benefit over commercialism.[8]

The fear of national decline and the focus on health at the individual level

The progress of the Public Health Movement failed to eradicate major health inequalities, a fact which became clear in the examination of Boer War recruits, 38% of whom were rejected as physically inadequate. Alleged physical, mental and moral deterioration of the British 'race' had been a concern since the 1880s, fuelled by the theories and solutions advanced by social Darwinists supported by the 'science' of eugenics –

the devising of policies to improve the genetic quality of the human race through selective breeding. The eugenicists opposed many of the reforms advanced by the Public Health Movement on the grounds that they encouraged survival and breeding among genetically 'degraded groups' (i.e. the poor).

To address these issues, a governmental committee was established in 1904, the Inter-Departmental Committee on Physical Deterioration, which concluded that there was no progressive deterioration of the 'race' and improvements in health were possible if there were changes in food, clothing, overcrowding, cleanliness, drunkenness and home management.[9]

As a result of the perceived failure of public health measures and the shift to the germ theory of disease, the focus moved from societal to individual responsibility for health.[4] Mothers were held mainly responsible for family health, as illustrated by evidence presented to the Inter-Departmental Committee on Physical Deterioration which, in many cases, focused on an apparent maternal indifference or maternal inefficiency (also *see* Chapter 8, p. 232).[4,10] Welfare and preventive health policies were geared to the concept of 'maternal inefficiency'; health visiting services, initially voluntary gentlewomen visitors, and child welfare and antenatal clinics were developed to educate mothers and eradicate inefficient maternal practices and improve hygiene. Educational initiatives complemented these preventive health developments: schools and continuing educational institutions were encouraged to offer 'social education' so that the foundations of maternal competence could be laid, and school boards started to lay greater emphasis on cookery, household management and child care.[9]

Against the trend of early 20th-century British social and welfare policy, many women's groups argued for material improvements, such as the mother's endowment demanded by the Fabian Women's Group, and free medical treatment for women and children, in addition to education in order to combat high levels of infant mortality.[9] These demands went unheeded but, partly as a result of the report of the Inter-Departmental Committee on Physical Deterioration, a school meals service was introduced in 1906 and a school medical service in 1907.[9]

National Health Insurance, the National Health Service and the Welfare State

The 1911 National Health Insurance (NHI) Act, introduced to 'keep up with the Germans', provided medical, sickness, disablement, maternity and sanatorium benefits to all manual workers aged over 16 years and earning below £160 per year.[4,9] Workers' weekly contributions assured various services: cash payments during sickness, medical treatment, including GP consultations, drugs and appliances but excluding hospital specialist consultations, and additional benefits offered by the Approved Societies through which the payments were administered. NHI did little for most married women and children when they were ill and Jones argues that the main concern of the Government was to maintain the physical efficiency of male breadwinners ([9] p. 27).

Prior to the inception of the NHS in July 1948, there had been moves towards the establishment of a comprehensive service, fuelled by the problems of caring for civilian casualites during the Second World War. The administration of hospital services had been regionalised and national direction was given by the Ministry of Health, initially established in 1919. Hospital services had been in crisis and in 1942 the Beveridge Report on Social Insurance and Allied Services recommended comprehensive health services. The reforming Labour administration introduced welfare benefits to maternity, unemployment and sickness as well as the NHS, which offered comprehensive 'free at the time of use' services. Subsequently other European countries have overtaken the British Welfare State, offering more comprehensive and more generous benefits for unemployment and social welfare. As in the USA and the rest of Europe, the last 20 years have seen a questioning of the welfare consensus, which survived well into the 1970s, and economic and social policies have eroded many of the welfare provisions offered in the 1950s and 1960s.

Social policies and health inequalities

Social policy in less developed countries

As discussed in Chapter 5 (p. 104), many less developed countries, such as China, Costa Rica and Sri Lanka, are high achievers in terms of health and human development despite low GNP per capita. Others, such as Brazil and Saudi Arabia, fail to achieve their expected health and human development levels despite being comparatively rich. The explanation for these differences in achievement seems to lie in social policy. The high achievers, though very different in many aspects, have demonstrated the political will to improve health outcomes for their populations, including the urban and rural poor. Their social policies include the reduction of inequalities of income distribution and ensuring relative equality of food distribution and availability. These countries have also addressed the issue of universal education, with particular emphasis on female literacy.

By contrast, richer countries, such as Brazil, have very marked inequality of income distribution, with abject poverty co-existing with extreme wealth. The street children of the major Brazilian cities stand as testimony to this phenomenon: the indifference and lack of political will is reflected in the brutal treatment of these children, who are products of the uncontrolled economic expansion of Brazil and its industrial cities.

International economic policies play an important role in shaping how less developed countries are able to respond to social and health inequalities. Colonial rule in many of these countries led to distortions of local food economies and land ownership which continue to be reflected in the production of cash crops for export at the expense of food production for local consumption.[11] Industrial production is frequently controlled by international conglomerates based in developed countries, reducing the power of government in less developed countries to regulate their activities. Marketing policies are equally difficult to control, as the baby milk controversy illustrates.[12]

In the 1970s, banks in developed countries embarked on massive loan programmes to less developed countries and the structural adjustment programmes (SAPs), imposed by the International Monetary Fund (IMF) and the World Bank on countries which got into serious debt as a consequence, restrict the freedom of governments to embark on social, health and education programmes aimed at tackling health inequalities.[13] SAPs have resulted in a fall in expenditure on health and education (though not military expenditure) in 'adjusted' countries, health service charges have been imposed, incomes have been reduced and food prices increased. For example, Uganda currently spends US$2.50 per head annually on health and US$15 per head on debt servicing[14] and there is evidence that adjustment tends to have a negative effect on food security at the household and national levels.[15] The precise effects of these programmes are disputed; however, there can be little doubt that the impact falls mainly on the poor, whose diet and access to education and health services are further restricted.[13-17]

As a result of the debt crisis and other factors, such as disadvantageous terms of trade, declining aid and national insecurity, gains made worldwide in health status over the last few decades are being lost in the poorest parts of the world with the result that the health of an increasing number of the world's poorest children is deteriorating.[18] Urgent measures are needed to halt this decline. The Jubilee 2000 campaign for the cancellation of US$160–300 billion debt to the 52 most heavily indebted countries has met with partial success;[14] an agreement was reached in autumn 1999 to write off US$60 billion debt owed by the 41 most indebted countries, and the UK government has announced its intention to write off all debts owed to the UK once countries start to receive help from the World Bank and the IMF under the Highly Indebted Poor Countries scheme.[19]

A good example of a high achieving state which has protected its poor against the worst effects of debt and international economic decline is Kerala State on the southwest coast of India. Kerala has resisted the temptation to follow other less developed countries which have tried to solve their problems of poverty and underdevelopment by boosting industrial production and investment in expensive technology, and has concentrated on land reform and access to public services.[20] Land reform has redistributed both wealth and power from a ruling elite to smallholders and landless peasants; public food distribution at controlled prices has ensured that even the poorest have an adequate subsistence diet; public health measures ensuring better housing, water, sanitation and immunisation and well-funded, accessible health services have made healthcare accessible to all; a long history of literacy programmes has ensured that literacy among the lowest castes is the highest in India.[20] Despite the recent threat of unemployment, the social policies of Kerala State are a convincing example of the possibilities of reducing health inequalities and improving health for all citizens, even in one of the world's poorest areas.

Kerala's success has been based on more equitable distribution of state resources. The appropriateness of this approach as a way of reducing the health effects of poverty is confirmed in a study based on World Bank figures which looks at the combined effect of growth and income inequality on poverty in less developed countries.[21] On average, a 10% growth rate reduced the poverty headcount (the percentage of people living on less than US$1 per day) by 9% in countries where income was reasonably well distributed. The same growth rate reduced the poverty headcount by only 3% in countries where income was less equally distributed. Growth alone is not the answer; it must be combined with social policies which ensure more equal distribution of the rewards of economic growth.

Social policy in developed countries

Land reform as practised in Kerala has little relevance to modern developed countries. However, social policies which seek to redistribute income and reduce income inequalities, as land reform does in Kerala, are of great relevance to health inequalities in developed countries.

A series of recent reports contrasting health status in different developed countries demonstrate that countries, such as the UK and the USA, pursuing social policies which increase income differentials between rich and poor have slower improvements in the health status of their population as a whole and widening health inequalities.[22-26] Life expectancy at birth for Japanese males increased from 63.6 in 1955 to 75.2 in 1986 compared with an increase from 67.5 to 71.9 for British males over the same time period.[22] Part of the explanation for the Japanese overtaking the British in life expectancy is that whilst income differentials between the highest and lowest income quintiles are increasing in the UK, they are decreasing in Japan. Economic growth rates are higher in Japan, unemployment is much lower and there has been a greater increase in the percentage of 20–24 year-olds in tertiary education.[24]

The Unicef reports show that the social health of children (measured as a combination of IMR, government spending on education, suicide rate among teenagers and income distribution) in some developed countries (UK, USA, Canada, New Zealand and Australia) declined whilst it continued to rise in others (Germany, France and the Scandinavian and Benelux countries).[23,24] The reports identify *laissez-faire*, market-driven social and economic policies which have led to higher levels of unemployment and lower wage rates, as one of the main reasons for the difference in performance. In addition, tax policies pursued in these countries have tended to shift from progressive taxation (basically redistributing income from rich to poor) to regressive taxation. Along with reductions in welfare benefits, this has resulted in the poor in all these countries becoming worse off, with 21% of children in the USA living in poverty, 9% in Canada, Britain and Australia and less than 5% in France, Germany, the Netherlands and Sweden (*see* also Chapter 2). Figure 10.1 shows the relation between relative poverty and IMR in these countries.

The consequences of recent social policy options can be seen within as well as between countries. Over the period 1981–91, mortality differentials between the most affluent and deprived areas in the northern region of England increased in all age categories.[27] Among men in the 15–44 age groups, mortality rated in the poorest areas showed an actual rise over the ten-year period. A similar widening of differentials was demonstrated in a study from Scotland examining mortality over the same time period.[28] A recently published book[29] documents the evidence for a widening gap in mortality and morbidity at all

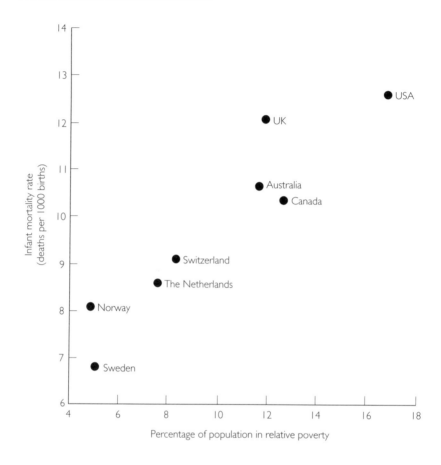

Figure 10.1   Relative poverty and IMR for eight OECD countries, 1980. (Source [26] p. 21)

ages between the most privileged and most deprived in the UK. The authors are unequivocal in linking the increasing health inequalities to increasing income inequalities, concluding 'had inequalities in health not been allowed to rise during the 1980s as a direct consequence of rising inequalities in income, then thousands of people would not have died prematurely'. ([29] p. 166) Pro-market reforms in New Zealand, similar to those introduced in the UK after 1979, were responsible for a decline in relative income among the Maori population which was followed by an increase in mortality ratios relative to the rest of the population.[30]

The social policy differences between countries, highlighted by the Unicef reports, give only a very broad picture of available social policy options and how they influence health. Examination of component parts of social policy will provide a more detailed picture and indicates important policy initiatives which can contribute to a reduction in health inequalities in developed countries. Much of the data are drawn from the UK and the USA, but comparisons are made with other countries where appropriate.

Employment

As a result of the world economic recession of the 1980s, unemployment in many industrialised countries has risen sharply. In 1985, it was estimated that over 35 million people were out of work in these countries.[31] The International Labor Office (ILO) estimated that there would be a global need for 1 billion additional jobs by the year 2000. The USA and the UK have seen particularly steep rises in unemployment, with a rise in the US unemployment rate from 3.5% in 1969 to 9.5% in 1983, and UK official figures rising to over 3 million (unofficial estimates were nearer 4 million) during the 1980s.[32] Young men are over-represented in these figures and, within cities, unemployment levels in this age group reached over 30% in the early 1990s.[33] Unemployment levels are closely linked to levels of child and family poverty (*see* Chapter 2, p. 40).

The effects of the world recession have been exacerbated in the UK and the USA by economic policies which have maintained artificially high interest rates and reduced government subsidies to traditional heavy industries, forcing them to close or cut back severely on employment. Since 1979, there has been a 36% fall in manufacturing jobs in the UK.[34] The result has been a shift towards low-paid part-time jobs, predominantly taken by women.

The newly elected UK government is committed to a policy of encouraging lone parents to come off benefits and undertake paid employment. Combined with the newly introduced Working Families Tax Credit, this is intended to raise large numbers of children in lone-parent families out of poverty. The lack of affordable child day care, however, is a major disincentive to paid work for lone parents in the UK.[35] In addition, there is evidence that if welfare recipients find only low-wage, stressful jobs, working may be counter-productive for the well-being of the family and the children.[36]

Incomes, taxation and public sector transfers

Wage rates in low income employment have been forced down as a result of labour market changes and high unemployment levels and deliberate government policy which has deregulated markets. In the USA, an increasing percentage of men aged between 25 and 54 do not earn enough to keep a family of four out of poverty.[32] Young men, particularly those in ethnic minority groups and those with limited education, are most likely to fall into this group of 'working poor'. The UK Conservative government insisted on staying outside the provisions of the European Union's Social Charter, designed to protect the rights of low-paid workers. The New Labour government elected in 1997 has introduced a minimum wage and accepted the Social Charter, but remains committed to many aspects of the unregulated labour market espoused by their predecessors.

Market-orientated governments have pursued a regressive taxation policy. Tax relief for the rich has been instituted with the result that in the USA the effective tax paid by the richest 5% has fallen by approximately one-fifth and that paid by the richest 1% by one-third over a 20-year period, and in the UK the tax burden of a married man with two children earning five times average earnings fell from 48.8% of gross earnings to 38.5% in the ten years from 1979 to 1989.[28] In the same period, the overall tax burden of those on average earnings rose from 35.1% to 37.3%. The promise of the UK Government to 'get government off our backs' seems to have worked only for a small section of the population. The expansion, since the mid-1980s, of the Earned Income Tax Credits in the USA has provided the largest cash assistance programme for families with children, lifting some of them out of poverty;[37] however, these changes have not been enough to offset the effects of other retrograde tax measures and the main burden has remained on the poor sections of the population.[32] Indirect taxation using value added tax (VAT) has represented an extra burden on the poor. These taxes are placed on purchases, and where these are essentials such as fuel and food, the load falls unevenly on the poor, who use a higher percentage of their income to purchase necessities.

Public sector transfers in the form of welfare and other benefits have been, along with taxation, the main mechanism by which income has been redistributed. The trend during most of the 20th century in long-established industrial countries, such as Britain and the USA, towards a shrinking share of aggregate wealth commanded by the richest 5% depended on these twin instruments of redistribution. Since the early 1980s, this trend has been reversed in the UK and the USA.[38]

In the UK, despite an overall rise in the social security budget since 1980, related directly to the rise in unemployment, individual welfare benefits have been reduced either by complex changes in the benefit system or by removing the link between benefits and the cost of living. Cash transfers in the USA have continued to rise but, since 1974, the rise has been solely in social insurance which mainly benefits the elderly; public assistance, mainly spent on welfare, housing, Medicaid and food stamps for those neither aged nor disabled, has been static despite the increased numbers of families with children in poverty.[32] The US federal Special Supplemental Food Program for Women, Infants and Children (WIC), created by the US Congress in 1972, has been under attack by market-orientated politicians and some paediatricians on the grounds that it encouraged the development of welfare dependency.[39] The results of an evaluation of WIC carried out on the government's behalf, showing that it had positive benefits for the health of women and children, were delayed and distorted in order to persuade government to discontinue the programme (*see* also Chapter 11, p. 320).[39,40]

Public sector transfers are intended both as a 'welfare safety net' and a mechanism for income redistribution. One measure of their success in redistributing income is the extent to which they ensure the economic well-being of the recipients. Table 10.1

Table 10.1 Economic welfare in families strongly depending on public transfers. (Source [41] Table 12)

Country	Proportion of families %	Economic well-being as a proportion of average %
Sweden	17.8	83.2
UK	14.2	48.3
West Germany	25.4	67.2
Norway	16.0	67.7
Canada	8.5	41.3
Israel	7.3	49.6
USA	9.5	39.9
Switzerland	4.5	51.9
Average	12.8	56.1

compares the economic welfare of families dependent on public sector transfers in different European countries.[41]

Sweden is by far the most successful in achieving the goal of income redistribution. The UK, Canada and the USA are the least successful. Tax and public sector transfers reduced the proportion of households with children living below half the median income (adjusted for family size) in Sweden from 17% to 2% but from 25% to only 22% in the USA (Figure 10.2).[40] Spending on income security is also negatively correlated with a country's proportion of children living in low income households (Figure 10.3).[40]

Labour market earnings for adults in households with children appear to be another important mechanism by which child poverty is reduced. Using data from the Luxembourg Income Study (the same data source as that used in Figures 10.2 and 10.3), Bradbury and Jantti[43] demonstrate that it is high labour market earnings of Swedish children that ensure high living standards for the most disadvantaged Swedish children. The UK, Australia and Canada are characterised by low labour market incomes and heavy reliance by low income families on social transfers. The authors postulate that the more rigid and

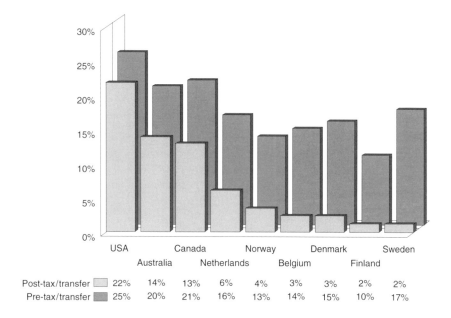

Figure 10.2   Low income rates among households with children: before and after taxes and transfers, circa 1991. Low income is measured using 50% median disposable income, adjusted for family size. (Source [42] p. 22)

regulated labour markets of the Scandinavian countries play an important part in protecting children from poverty.[43]

As a result of the changes in taxation and public sector transfers, the gap between rich and poor in some countries has increased. The poorest 5% of families in the UK experienced a fall in income before taking account of housing costs between 1979 and 1991, compared with the richest 5% whose income rose by 58%.[44] Comparing rich and poor parts of the south-western English city of Bristol (one of the richest cities in the country), Townsend and co-workers found that there had been a decline in car ownership in the poorest areas compared with a marked rise in the richest areas.[45] Electricity disconnections and free school meals, markers of material deprivation, had increased in the poorest areas but declined in the richest areas. Incomes for the poorest US families have grown at a slower rate than those for the richest.[46]

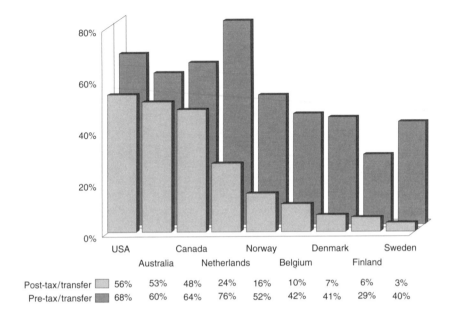

Figure 10.3 International comparison of spending on income security and children's low income rates, circa 1991. Low income is measured using 50% median disposable income, adjusted for family size. (Source [42] p. 25)

Other elements of social policy relevant to health

Housing is one of the potent mechanisms by which poverty is linked to health (*see* Chapter 9, p. 244). Alongside changes in British welfare and taxation policies in the 1980s there has been a marked change in the provision of social housing. Government spending on housing fell from £13.1 billion in 1979 to £5.8 billion in 1992.[47] At the same time, a policy of sale of social houses to sitting tenants realised £28 billion for local councils by the end of 1993 but government regulations prohibited the use of these monies to improve the social housing stock. As a result there has been a general deterioration in public housing and an increase in homelessness, with the number of households with children officially homeless in 1992 reaching

170 000. These families are expensively housed in overcrowded and insanitary hotels.

Recognising the well-documented links between housing and health inequalities (*see* also Chapter 9, p. 244), Best, as part of an overall agenda for action to tackle health inequalities, lists a number of national policy initiatives aimed at reducing health inequalities through improved housing.[48] These include: targeted investment in new and improved social housing; spending of existing housing subsidies to better effect – currently in the UK owner-occupiers receive more subsidy than renters; an investment programme to improve heating and insulation, which are poor in many UK houses; investment in community development in disadvantaged neighbourhoods.

Alongside these national initiatives, there is a need for policy to encourage local initiatives based on community participation. Ineichen describes the development of the Eldon Street Community Association in Liverpool which, against enormous economic and social odds, has become the largest housing cooperative in the UK and has developed community businesses and social care networks.[6] Given a favourable national policy such initiatives would be able to flourish, with the added advantage that the local people have a genuine stake in the success of the project.

Education policy has an important bearing on health (*see* Chapter 9, p. 247). There is evidence that the UK government's attempts to make schools more efficient and shift the burden of educational expenditure to a local level have resulted in a fall in educational standards, which particularly affects the least able pupils in some of the most deprived inner-city schools.[49] The result is an inevitable widening of the gap between privileged and deprived, clearly reflected in the decline in reading age differentially affecting the most deprived children which has been noted in the UK in the 1980s.[26] The fact that these differences in performance between deprived and privileged are not immutable comes from various other developed countries which have succeeded in overcoming this differential; for example, the close relation of British children's mathematics scores to their parents' occupational class is not seen in Japan, where no occupational trend was noted in the International Maths Test among 11-year-olds.[26]

The importance of the causal debate in determining social policy

It was my express intention in writing this book to take a historical and global view of poverty and child health. As can be seen from the preceding chapters, a vein of political controversy runs through the history of research and social policy related to poverty and health. Ever since the days of Chadwick and Villerme (*see* Chapter 4, p. 79), a fierce debate has been fought out intellectually and politically centring on the determinants of poverty and its health effects: they broadly divide into the individualist, behavioural 'culture of poverty' and the societal, materialist 'structure determines behaviour' schools of thought (*see* Part Three). These opposing explanations and social policy options have been advanced in all countries, developed where absolute poverty is rare and less developed where it is widespread, and in all historical periods, since the problem became recognised.

Thus, the causal debate is not an esoteric intellectual exercise, conducted in academic circles and through the pages of academic journals, divorced from the experience of ordinary citizens; it is of immediate and long-term relevance to the well-being of millions globally, particularly women and children, who are most affected by social policy changes. In this context, it is useful to explore how current important social policy choices reflect the theoretical debates which underlie them.

The drive to reduce and limit public cash transfers and reverse the trend to redistribution from rich to poor in some developed countries has been accompanied and underpinned by a modern version of the long-standing debate. In direct line of continuity with the individualist explanations for poverty and health differences advanced around the turn of the 20th century with additional eugenicist echoes, individual and moral failings and behaviours rather than structurally determined social conditions are seen as the main reason for the growing social exclusion of the poor. A dependency culture, it is argued, has developed as a result of welfare benefit provision, with consequent sapping of individual enterprise and the necessity to work. Linked with the dependency culture is the discovery of an 'underclass' (*see* also Chapter 8) made up of those chronically dependent on welfare, with a particular focus on young lone mothers.

These theories have been developed particularly by Charles Murray, a conservative social scientist; he argues that poverty has largely been caused by the availability of financial support from outside families because if starvation were the only alternative, people would work.[50] These ideas, with their resonances back to the New Poor Law in 19th-century Britain, underpinned Reaganite social policies and the 1988 US Family Support Act, which curtailed public support for lone mothers and withdrew it from claimants who set up independent households before they reached the age of 18. Murray has argued that single mothers in Britain are wreaking havoc on society by forsaking 'traditional family values'.[50] The proposed social policy initiatives to deal with this group, who are seen as the basis of the underclass, involve a return to the stigma of unmarried parenthood and enforced adoption and admission of the children into orphanages, in the same way as the workhouses of 19th- and early 20th-century Britain were used to house and discipline illegitimate children and their mothers (*see* above). Teenage mothers have been attacked for getting themselves pregnant in order to be given a home ([51] p. 197) but the available evidence does not support this contention. As Leach points out:

> *Babies-for-gain are a myth and a myth without foundation as there is no gain; even in Norway, the country which through its 'transitional benefit' provides most generously for women rearing children as their sole parents, the total package of entitlements enables them to avoid poverty but does not maintain them at a level as high as that enjoyed by two-parent families.* ([51] p. 198)

Attempts have been made to define the 'underclass' for scientific purposes.[52] The definitions fall broadly into persistent poverty-based, behaviour-based and location-based measures.[50] These differing definitions clearly reflect the causal debate and do not represent a real advance of knowledge about poverty itself or the reasons for the recent trend towards children, families and lone parents as the main groups in poverty in all developed countries, independent of welfare policies (*see* Chapter 2, p. 43). Unsurprisingly, whichever measure of the underclass is used, the groups so defined show considerable overlap and all contain disproportionate numbers of minority ethnic groups, poorly educated adults and individuals living in inner-city neighbourhoods.[52]

The assumptions underlying the social policy options flowing from theories of the underclass and the dependency culture have been supported by medical academics such as George Graham, a professor of nutrition and paediatrics at Johns Hopkins University, who argues that the real problem is not poverty and inadequate dietary intake but the promiscuous behaviour of poor mothers and related 'social cancers'.[39]

A UK research programme, the DHSS/SSRC Joint Working Party on Transmitted Deprivation, which extended over the ten years between 1972 and 1982, was established to explore the idea that deprivation is transmitted across generations by cultural and psychological processes within the family. The programme was initiated by Sir Keith Joseph, the then Secretary of State for Social Services in the Conservative Government and later one of the main Thatcherite ideologues, essentially in pursuit of the same explanation of persistent poverty as Murray. However, as Brown records:

> It was gradually acknowledged on the programme that structural factors as well as personal factors must play a part in both the generation and the transmission of deprivation. ([42] p. 2)

She concludes from the research progamme set up to explore the opposite view:

> Social structure creates and sustains social disadvantage. The bulk of deprivation suffered in society arises

out of the systematic disadvantage of vulnerable groups. Vulnerable groups are disadvantaged by their position in society, above all by their class position. ([53] p. 11)

Brown argues that solutions to the transmission of deprivation cannot be found in the outstanding individuals who do break out of their social class, as the upward movement of individuals does not lead to a change of position of whole groups and:

Individuals may succeed against the odds but the odds don't change because of isolated success stories. ([53] p. 12)

The programme supported social policies aimed at reducing basic occupational inequalities which would influence income, health, educational and housing inequalities. The fact that so little evidence has been found in the Transmitted Deprivation project, and others before it, to support the existence of a significant group of undeserving poor or 'underclass' prompted Shaw and co-workers to make the following scathing comment:

In the history of scientific endeavour, there cannot be many more thoroughly falsified theories than the undeserving poor argument in Britain. There is more evidence for the existence of the Loch Ness Monster than for the existence of a homogeneous group of people who form an 'underclass' in the United Kingdom. Huge amounts of money and scientific effort have been wasted over the past 150 years in unsuccessfully hunting for the undeserving poor in Britain. They simply do not exist in sufficient numbers to justify the effort or any comprehensive arguments based on their existence. ([29] p. 206)

A UK social and economic policy vision for children

The Acheson Report,[54] commissioned by the UK Labour Government in 1997 as an independent inquiry into health inequalities, recommended that a high priority be given to policies aimed at improving health and reducing health inequalities in women of child-bearing age, expectant mothers and young children by promoting the material support of parents. The recommendations of the Inquiry,[55] and the subsequent policy responses of the UK Government,[29] have been criticised on the grounds that they avoid the key issue of redistribution through progressive taxation. Taxation changes, such as the introduction of Children's Tax Credit and the introduction of the 10p income tax band, were intended to ensure 'redistribution by stealth' – in other words, redistribution without increasing the income tax take from the rich. These changes, plus the rash of initiatives designed to focus health and social services on the most needy (Health Action Zones, Sure Start and others), are unlikely to be effective in reversing the inequalities which have occurred over the last two decades and to achieve the Government's expressed objective of eliminating child poverty within 20 years.[29] The budgetary changes introduced in 1999 have been shown to leave 98% of the poorest families unaffected, with poor families with children gaining at the expense of poor families without children.[29]

Shaw *et al.*[29] propose an alternative social and economic policy vision based on the principle that the poor have too little money and the solution to ending poverty is to provide them with more money. They state: 'the quickest and most cost-effective method of alleviating poverty is to increase the value of welfare benefits and pensions and improve public services and social housing' (p. 191). They support an economic and social policy, as outlined by Leach, based on the starting point of ensuring that every child is 'rich enough' because:

> ... *poverty in childhood has such heavy long-term costs that money spent to prevent it would yield far*

better returns than extant welfare policies; that any
extra costs incurred, over and above current budgets,
would be apparent rather than real, and that focusing
on children would ultimately produce more caring
and creative societies. ([51] p. 187)

Reflecting a similar response to the current dilemmas and
shortcomings of social policy, Basic Income Schemes have been
proposed which provide a minimum income, the amount of
which is based only on age and family status but is otherwise
unconditional.[29,56,57]

Shaw and co-workers ([29] pp. 199–200) proposed the adoption
of the following social policies to reduce health inequalities
amongst UK children:

- All pregnant women should be able to afford an adequate
  diet. The current maternity allowance is insufficient to
  achieve this aim and should be increased, particularly for
  women dependent on Income Support and/or in low-paid
  jobs.

- Additional benefits are required to support families with
  children as the rates are currently so low that families with
  children will eventually sink into poverty if they become
  dependent on Income Support for any length of time.

- As approximately 25% of all children are born to mothers
  under 25 years old, the current supposition that people
  under 25 years require lower rates of benefit than those
  over 25 should be urgently re-examined.

- Additional benefits for lone parents are needed to reflect
  the additional financial and time costs of caring as a lone
  parent compared with two-parent families.

- Universal child benefit rates should be increased beyond
  the levels proposed in the 1999 budget.

In view of the disincentive to employment among lone parents
and low income mothers in the UK resulting from the lack
of adequate day care, considered above,[35] an additional social

policy of key importance would be the provision of affordable and universally available day care for children.

A social and economic policy vision for the world's children

Building on the Declaration of the March 1995 World Summit for Social Development, which recommended a vision of social, economic and political inclusion and a recognition of economic growth as a means not an end in itself, Save the Children Fund propose a children's agenda for the future, the main features of which are as follows:[58]

- an economic model which is inclusive and allows everyone in society to secure access to a sustainable livelihood and participate fully in the benefits of economic and social progress

- measures which ensure that children's needs, rights and perspectives are respected, including recognising each society's responsibility to give children an equal start in life, investing in children, developing child-specific information and increasing child participation in decisions affecting their lives

- measures which enable adults to combine their child care and productive roles effectively

- investment of tax revenues in child care and child development

- additional resources for female literacy and education

- reform of legal frameworks to protect and promote the best interests of children as outlined in the UN Convention on the Rights of the Child.

Summary

1   Social policy decisions have a major impact on child poverty and health.

2   Neo-liberal, monetarist economic and social policies pursued in developed countries, such as the UK and the USA, in recent years have been responsible for increasing child poverty and exacerbating its health consequences.

3   Imposed on less developed debtor countries, the effects of these same policies have fallen particularly on the poor, with long-term consequences for child health and development.

4   Countries, developed and less developed, which have pursued social policies aimed at reducing income disparity and supporting the poor and vulnerable have succeeded in reducing poverty and its health consequences.

5   There is a strong case for child-centred policies which aim to give all children an equal start in life – the long-term benefits of such policies are likely to far outweigh the short-term costs.

References

1   Wise P and Meyers A (1988) Poverty and child health. *Pediatr. Clin. North Am.* 35:1169–86.

2   Waterson A (1995) How can child health services contribute to a reduction in health inequalities in childhood? In *Progress in Community Child Health, Vol. 1* (ed. NJ Spencer). Churchill Livingstone, Edinburgh.

3   Benzeval M, Judge K and Whitehead M (eds) (1995) *Tackling Inequalities in Health: An Agenda for Action*. King's Fund, London.

4   Webster C (ed.) (1993) *Caring for Health: History and Diversity*. Open University Press, Milton Keynes.

5   Scott J (1994) *Poverty and Wealth: Citizenship, Deprivation and Privilege*. Longman, London.

6   Ineichen B (1993) *Homes and Wealth: How Housing and Health Interact*. EFN Spon, London.

7   Haynes B (1991) *Working Class Life in Victorian Leicester: the Joseph Dare Reports.* Leicester County Council, Leicester.

8   Lowry S (1991) *Housing and Health.* BMJ Publications, London.

9   Jones H (1994) *Health and Society in Twentieth Century Britain.* Longman, London.

10 Smith D and Nicholson M (1992) Poverty and ill health: controversies past and present. *Proc. Roy. Coll. Phys. Edinburgh.* **22**:190–9.

11 Gray A (ed.) (1993) *World Health and Disease.* Open University Press, Milton Keynes.

12 War on Want (1975) *The Baby Killer.* War on Want, London.

13 Costello A, Watson F and Woodward D (1994) *Human Faces or Human Facade? Adjustment and the Health of Mothers and Children.* Centre for International Child Health, Institute of Child Health, London.

14 Abbasi K (1999) Free the slaves. *BMJ.* **318**:1568–9.

15 Woodward D (1992) *Debt, adjustment and food security.* Save the Children Overseas Department Working Paper No. 3, Save the Children, London.

16 Godlee F (1993) Third world debt. *BMJ.* **307**:1369–70.

17 World Bank (1993) *World Development Report 1993: Investing in Health.* Oxford University Press, New York.

18 Save the Children (1998) *The Save the Children Fund (UK) Global Health Sector Strategy.* Save the Children, London.

19 *The Guardian*, Saturday 18th December, 1999.

20 Franke RW and Chasin BH (1992) Kerala State, India: radical reform as development. *Int. J. Health Serv.* **22**:139–56.

21 Hanmer L (1999) Are the DAC targets achievable? Poverty and human development in the year 2015. *J. Int. Develop.* 2:547–63.

22 Marmot MG and Smith GD (1989) Why are the Japanese living longer? *BMJ.* **299**:1547–51.

23 Unicef (1993) *The Progress of Nations.* Unicef, New York.

24 Hewlett SA (1993) *Child Neglect in Rich Nations.* Unicef, New York.

25 Power C (1994) Health and social inequality in Europe. *BMJ.* **308**:1153–6.

26 Wilkinson RG (1994) *Unfair Shares: The Effects of Widening Income Differences on the Welfare of the Young.* Barnados Publications, Ilford.

27 Phillimore P, Beattie A and Townsend P (1994) Widening health inequalities in northern England. *BMJ.* **308**:1125–8.

28 McLoone P and Boddy FA (1994) Deprivation and mortality in Scotland, 1981 and 1991. *BMJ.* **309**:1465–70.

29 Shaw M, Dorling D, Gordon D *et al.* (1999) *The Widening Gap: Health Inequality and Policy in Britain.* The Policy Press, University of Bristol, Bristol.

30 Brown MC (1999) Policy-induced changes in Maori mortality patterns in the New Zealand economic reform period. *Health Econom.* **8**:127–36.

31 Westcott G, Svensson PG and Zollner HFK (1985) *Health Policy Implications of Unemployment.* WHO Regional Office for Europe, Copenhagen.

32 Danziger S and Stern J (1990) *The causes and consequences of child poverty in the United Kingdom.* Innocenti Occasional Papers, No. 10. Unicef International Child Development Centre, Florence, Italy.

33   Sheffield Health Authority (1991) *Healthcare and disease: a profile of Sheffield.* Sheffield Health Authority, Sheffield.

34   Walker R (1995) Families, poverty and work. *Centre for Research in Social Policy Briefing.* 6:1.

35   Bradshaw J, Kennedy S, Kilkey M *et al.* (1996) *The Employment of Lone Parents: A Comparison of Policies in 20 Countries.* Family Policy Studies Centre, London.

36   Parcel TL and Menaghan EG (1997) Effects of low-wage employment on family well-being. *The Future of Children.* 7:116–21.

37   Plotnick RD (1997) Child poverty can be reduced. *The Future of Children.* 7:72–87.

38   Townsend P (1994) The rich man in his castle. *BMJ.* 309: 1674–5.

39   Brown JL, Gershoff SN and Cook JT (1992) The politics of hunger: when science and ideology clash. *Int. J. Health Serv.* 22:221–37.

40   Rush D, Alvir J, Johnson KS *et al.* (1988) The National WIC Evaluation: evaluation of the special supplemental food program for women, infants and children. *Am J. Clin. Nutr.* 48:412–28.

41   Aguiler R and Gustafsson B (1988) *Public Sector Transfers and Income Taxes. An International Comparison with Micro Data.* Department of Economics, University of Goteborg, Goteborg.

42   Ross DP, Scott K and Kelly M (1996) *Child Poverty: What are the Consequences?* Centre for International Statistics, Canadian Council on Social Development, Ottawa, Canada.

43   Bradbury B and Jantti M (1999) *Child poverty across industrialized nations.* Innocenti Occasional Papers, Economic and Social Policy Series No. 71. Unicef International Child Development Centre, Florence.

44   Goodman A and Webb S (1994) *For Richer, For Poorer*. Institute for Fiscal Studies, London.

45   Townsend P, Davidson N and Whitehead M (1992) *Inequalities in Health: The Black Report and the Health Divide*. Penguin, Harmondsworth.

46   US Congressional Budget Office (1988) *Trends in family income: 1970–86*. US Government Printing Office, Washington DC.

47   Heath I (1994) The poor man at his gate. *BMJ*. **309**:1685–6.

48   Best R (1995) The housing dimension. In *Tackling Inequalities in Health: an Agenda for Action* (eds M Benzeval, K Judge and M Whitehead). King's Fund, London.

49   Kumar V (1993) *Poverty and Inequality in the UK: The Effects on Children*. National Children's Bureau, London.

50   Murray C, Field F, Brown JC *et al*. (1990) *The Emerging British Underclass*. Institute of Economic Affairs Health and Welfare Unit, London.

51   Leach P (1994) *Children First*. Michael Joseph, London.

52   Mincy RB, Sawhill IV and Wolf D (1990) The underclass: definition and measurement. *Science*. **248**:450–3.

53   Brown M (ed.) (1983) *The Structure of Disadvantage*. Heinemann Educational Books, London.

54   Department of Health (1998) *Independent Inquiry into Inequalities in Health (The Acheson Report)*. The Stationery Office, London.

55   Davey Smith G, Shaw M and Dorling D (1998) The independent inquiry into inequalities in health. *BMJ*. **317**: 1465–6.

56   Desai M (1998) A basic income proposal. In *The State of the Future* (eds R Skidelsky, W Eltis, E Davis *et al*.). Social Market Foundation, London.

57   Bartley M (1994) Health costs of social injustice. *BMJ*. **309**:1177–8.

58   Save the Children Fund (1995) *Towards a Children's Agenda: New Challenges for Social Development*. Save the Children, London.

11

Innovative health service approaches and future research directions

Introduction

Health service interventions play a relatively small part in the response to health inequalities.[1] A range of social policy interventions seem to have more powerful effects on the reduction of poverty and its health consequences. However, health service interventions should not be either belittled or ignored: health services can alleviate and ameliorate the worst effects of poverty and are an important part of intersectoral approaches to health.[2-4]

Given the relatively minor role played by health service interventions, it may seem inappropriate that these are the subject of the penultimate chapter of this book. This book is written by a paediatrician with child health professionals as the main audience. I do not want those of them who read this book to leave it with the feeling that the health services in which they work and their day-to-day practice have no influence on the health of children living in poverty and that their particular contribution is of no real value. This chapter is written precisely because I want to stress the potential for health professionals and health services to influence policy and ensure equitable access of poor families to child health services, and to convince child health academics of the importance of research in this aspect of child health which, at least in the UK and the USA, has been given scant attention. For this reason, this chapter is in a sense the logical conclusion of the book, with its direct challenge for child health professionals to participate in service interventions aimed at reducing inequalities and the effects of poverty on the health of children.

In this chapter, the basic principles underlying effective health service interventions directed at reducing and alleviating health inequalities are considered first, followed by examples of international, national and local interventions which illustrate these principles in practice. Finally the chapter addresses future research directions.

Basic principles

Ever since the relationship between poverty and health was recognised, interventions designed to alleviate the worst effects of poverty on the health of children and mothers have been carried out. Many of these have ended in failure as they were based on wrong or ill thought-out principles. Recent examples are infant feeding programmes in Atlantic Canada,[5] aimed at reducing inequities but which result in stigmatisation of families. Most of the programmes adopt a family substitution role in the lives of children and function in a way that excludes parental participation. Experience in the USA has led to the adoption of a series of basic principles on which community initiatives should be based:[6] comprehensive (addressing many issues at once); coordinated, integrated and collaborative; accountable; flexible; preventive; family and community focused; participative; building on community strengths; responsive to individual difference; universally available. These and others are considered in more detail below.

Equity

If the poor are excluded from services either by financial or geographical constraints or services delivered to more affluent areas are better equipped and staffed (*see* Chapter 9, p. 251), such services will continue to perpetuate health inequalities. Equity of service provision must be an essential principle of successful interventions. As the WHO Health for All (HFA) 2000 initiative states: 'Health for all implies equity'. Even in a service established on the principle of equity such as the British National Health Service, there is a need for change to ensure equitable service delivery; Benzeval and co-workers suggest that much greater effort is needed to assess whether the NHS is achieving equal access for equal need for all social groups.[1] They recommend that local health services set up equity audits to monitor progress. The importance of equity audits are highlighted by a recent Scottish study of waiting times for cardiac surgery, which showed that socio-economically deprived patients are thought more likely to develop coronary health disease but are less likely to be investigated and offered surgery once it has developed.[7]

Empowerment and participation

In 1991, the *Daily Mail*, a conservative daily paper in Britain, gave its opinion of the *Health of the Nation* consultative paper as follows: 'As history shows, a determination to do good to people, whether they like it or not, is the basis of the most tyrannical behaviour by governments, whether on a petty or a major scale'. This book has taken an opposite view but it is important to recognise that well-meaning interventions made without the involvement of the recipients are always in danger of being viewed negatively. Experience in less developed countries as well as poorer areas of developed countries has led to widespread recognition of the need for community participation in interventions aimed at health gain. Participation is closely allied to empowerment, by which the participants become actively involved in changing their own life situation. Participation alone cannot overcome all the barriers to health arising from economic and social deprivation but, given a positive climate created by an equitable social policy, communities can become empowered to improve the health of their households.

Intersectoral working

Health service interventions alone are limited in their capacity to provide the conditions for reducing health inequalities.

Cooperation with a wide range of other agencies and sectors will enable interventions to be more effective. This approach has been developed through the WHO HFA 2000 programme and the Healthy Cities initiative which grew out of it.[8] The WHO Healthy Cities initiative, involving networks of over 1000 cities and towns throughout more than 27 countries in Europe, has been incorporated into the WHO Social Determinants Programme and is based on commitment to healthy public policy, partnerships for health and empowerment.[8] Intersectoral working needs to be facilitated actively with mechanisms, national and local, for ensuring that it is instituted and sustained. In addition to working together, agencies not traditionally concerned with health should assess on a regular basis the short- and long-term health impacts of their policy decisions. In Sweden, all national public agencies are required to report on specific goals to reduce socio-economic inequalities and analyse the health impact of all national policies.[9]

Information and data monitoring

Health inequalities cannot be tackled if data are inadequate to monitor trends. Some countries, such as Australia, have little history of routine data collection related to health in different socio-economic groups; as Jolly suggests, this may result from concerns about confidentiality and the perception of Australia as a classless society.[10] Britain has a long history of collecting occupation-based health data which have proved invaluable in exploring trends and patterns of health inequality. Disquiet has been expressed at the recent tendency for direct government control of health inequalities and poverty data and the potential for suppression of embarrassing statistics.[11] The newly elected Conservative Government attempted to undermine the impact of the Black Report in 1980; the report was not properly printed and the then Minister of Health wrote a dismissive foreword questioning the validity of the conclusions.[12]

Of equal importance to adequate national and local data are the parameters used to measure socio-economic status. Occupational class measures inadequately reflect SES differences and alternative measures are now being developed which better reflect health differentials between social groups (*see* Chapter 1 and Chapter 6).[13] This is particularly important in the monitoring of health inequalities among women and children.[14]

Information collection must include scientifically valid evidence of the effectiveness of interventions to reduce health inequalities.[4] An evidence-based approach will be an essential basis for influencing policy decisions.

Advocacy

It may appear to many that the health professions have been concerned exclusively with the treatment and care of individual patients. However, there is a long tradition of advocacy for individuals and groups of people which goes back as far as the birth of the Public Health Movement in the 19th century. Even when empowered, children and people living in poor social conditions need assistance with publicising their situation and creating the conditions for change. Health professionals are ideally placed to provide this advocacy and those committed to reducing health inequalities should seek to become skilled in this aspect of their work, which can be as powerful as any medication in combating ill health and disease. Advocacy for children has become linked solely with the protection of children from the violence of society and their own families. The advocacy proposed here focuses much more on the presentation of data related to poverty and child health and the advancement of policy solutions which promote child health, as well as the critique of policies which undermine the struggle for health.

Accessibility and availability

Closely linked with the equitable delivery of health services are the concepts of accessibility and availability. On a global scale, available and accessible health services are at a premium and it is the rural poor, often the majority of the population, to whom services are not readily available and for whom accessibility is the greatest problem. Most developed countries have services which are universally available, though access may be limited more by financial constraints than geography (*see* Chapter 9, p. 251).

However, there are other more subtle ways in which the access of people in more deprived areas can be impeded. Service-based interventions to reduce health inequalities need to specifically address these issues with service users: professionals can often assume that their services are readily available and accessible but unrecognised barriers prevent their proper use by disadvantaged families.[15] Participation and empowerment (*see* above) should facilitate this process, allowing communities to become part of the intervention design and ensuring that issues such as availability are adequately addressed.

Acceptability and relevance

Professional constructions of the determinants of health may differ from lay constructions, especially in situations where the population being served has different cultural traditions from the health professionals. Unacceptable services become inaccessible and unavailable. Services seen as irrelevant to local needs will not be used. Acceptability and relevance can only be assured through participation of the community in the development of services and empowering communities to modify and design interventions. These take on particular importance when interventions to reduce health inequalities are being considered.

Flexibility

Health services have traditionally been run for the convenience of the professionals and staff and not the clients. Flexibility of service provision is important in attempting to overcome health inequalities. For example, disadvantaged groups are more likely to need domiciliary or mobile services which increase access and availability and may prove more acceptable. Flexibility requires that health professionals and service managers and planners are able to adapt interventions to the needs of the children and their families.

Needs-driven interventions

Service provision in many countries has developed in a haphazard fashion with little relationship to any measure of need. Need can be variously defined but needs assessment measures have been developed which attempt to translate unmet health needs into service provision. As Benzeval and co-workers point out, resource allocation changes are required 'to ensure that all resources are allocated to areas in relation to their need for them' ([1] p. xxiii). A needs-driven service approach will lead naturally to interventions which reduce health inequalities.

Interventions which reflect some of these principles

The following examples of interventions designed to reduce child health inequalities have been chosen to demonstrate the application of the above principles in developed and less developed countries. Internationally initiated interventions are considered first, followed by national, local and, finally, individual practice level interventions.

International interventions

WHO and Unicef have initiated a series of interventions designed to improve health outcomes for poor children in less developed countries. Although some, such as the Oral Rehydration Treatment (ORT) programme described below, have been criticised on the grounds that they fail to tackle the underlying problem of safe water, these programmes have been enthusiastically adopted in some countries with some success. Nearly 1.6 million people globally are estimated to be at risk of iodine deficiency, and maternal iodine deficiency is estimated to be responsible for 30 000 stillbirths per year and more than 120 000 children born with hypothyroidism. Milder levels of deficiency are probably responsible for loss of intellectual potential in many children, with all its resultant consequences. Children in poor areas of poor countries are differentially affected.[16] Interventions in two countries are notable: in Syria, where the Ministry of Industry has a monopoly of salt production, iodine is now added as a supplement to the nation's salt; in Bolivia, where many small-scale salt producers operate, a private company has been established to popularise iodized salt, and the consequent growth in demand has been assisted by government intervention to maintain low prices.

Safe water is an acute problem in many rapidly growing cities in less developed countries. The population of Tagucigalpa, the capital of Honduras, has trebled in 20 years; many live in shanty towns known as *barrios marginales*. Water was unsafe and expensive, costing ten times as much as that for residents connected to the public water system. With Unicef's help, the Honduran National Water and Sanitation Agency launched a programme based on community participation in elected community water boards in each *barrio*, in which independent wells were sunk and communal tanks constructed. Within five years, 50 000 people in 26 *barrios* were getting safe water at the same time as cutting the annual household water bill from 40% to 4% of income.

ORT has been one of WHO/Unicef's most publicised and extensive campaigns, directed at more effective home-based management of diarrhoeal diseases which cause havoc in many less developed countries (*see* Chapter 5). Early childhood diarrhoea picks out poor children living in poor conditions with unsafe water. The ORT programme's progress in Egypt illustrates the possibilities and problems of health interventions which involve the health services.[16] In 1983, the Egyptian Government, supported by the US Agency for International Development, launched an ORT promotion campaign. Within two years, 96% of mothers were aware of ORT and usage rates were higher than 50%, contributing to the fall in IMR from 136/1000 in 1985 to 72/1000 in 1991. However, a combination of loss of external funding and prescribing of drug treatment by the medical profession undermined the programme. Recent WHO surveys indicate that ORT was used in 23% of cases and prescribed drugs in 54%.

The three examples considered above illustrate the potential of internationally initiated programmes. They confirm the importance of intersectoral working and the difficulties of relying on one sector, such as health, to carry out the programme. Community involvement in the process was vital to the success of the Honduran project, which was based on an alliance between government departments and local community-based organisations; by contrast, the lack of involvement of key personnel and local organisations seems to have contributed to the failure of the ORT programme in Egypt. The success of the Syrian and Bolivian projects was dependent on sensitivity to, and awareness of, local conditions.

National interventions

Early childhood education and enhanced development are associated with better health outcomes for poor children in less developed (*see* Chapter 5) and developed countries (*see* Chapter 6). Building on an experiment in a small fishing village, La Playa, the Colombian Government in 1987 embarked on a national programme of preschool provision which is founded in a community-participation model.[17] The programme now reaches over 1 million children at a cost of US$90 per child per year.

Save the Children, as an international non-governmental organisation (NGO), has initiated a Marginalised Youth Programme in a disadvantaged community in Jamaica, which, with the cooperation of the Jamaican Government, will be extended nationally.[17] The programme aims to enhance the self-esteem of children and parents by providing training and helping them to return to the regular school system. Informal street schools were used to initiate the programme and parental involvement was assured through a parenting group. The programme has had a major impact in the community, with knock-on effects on school attendance and local crime statistics, as well as providing a focus for the development of other community initiatives such as a shared day-care facility developed by the parents' group.

Tackling health inequalities at a national level requires a political commitment to change. A framework for change has been developed in the UK, but the 1992 Health of the Nation strategy specifically avoided any reference or commitment to equity and reduction of inequalities.[1,18] A task group was set up by the Department of Health to look at what were rather coyly referred to as 'health variations'; they recommended that the Department of Health should work in alliance with other government departments to encourage social policies which promote health as well as a programme of research related to 'health variations'.[19] They further recommended that health authorities and primary care purchasers should have plans for identifying and tackling variations and should monitor access to services to ensure equity.[19] The new UK government, elected in 1997, has acknowledged the importance of tackling health inequalities in the 'Our Healthier Nation' strategy[20] and in subsequent policy documents.[21,22] However, many of the proposed initiatives aimed at reducing health inequalities have been criticised as inadequate to the task (*see* also Chapter 10).[23]

The Australian Government has devised national strategies for tackling health inequalities.[24] The approach is two-pronged: specific targets are set for disadvantaged population groups and intersectoral proposals made to change key health determinants beyond the health sector. Proposals related to key determinants include improving overall adult literacy, employment, housing and providing a 'healthy environment'. Table 11.1 shows an example of goals and targets related to adequate housing as a key element of providing a healthy environment.

In the Netherlands a different approach has been taken.[25] Until 1980, health inequalities were unrecognised in post-war Netherlands. Prompted by the findings of the Black Report in the UK and the inclusion of targets for the reduction of health inequalities in the WHO HFA 2000 programme, renewed scientific interest developed from which a proposal for a major five-year coordinated research programme was formulated.[12,26] The programme was launched in 1989 with government funding. The programme aimed to increase knowledge of inequalities and their causes and influence health policy. Although the impact on policy is difficult to judge at this stage, national, regional and local initiatives have arisen from the programme, including an intersectoral working group at national level to

Table 11.1 Health environments: goals and targets developed as part of the Australian programme to reduce health inequalities. (Source [24] p. 784)

Goals and targets have been developed in six separate sectors covering the physical environmental (global pollution, air, water and soil contamination, indoor environment); housing, homes and community infrastructure; transport; work and the workplace; schools and healthcare settings.

An example: adequate housing

Goal: To increase the number of people living in adequate housing.

Proposed targets:

- priority population – Aboriginal and Torres Strait islanders in rural communities and settlements
- to reduce exposure to risks to health associated with poor living conditions.

Intermediate indicator – to increase the proportion of Aboriginal and Torres Strait islanders living in remote and rural communities who live in dwellings which have:

- potable water for drinking/cooking
- adequate water supply
- electricity
- bathing and laundry facilities
- sewage disposal facilities
- waste disposal
- adequate drainage.

Baseline – to be derived from ATSIC study into housing and community infrastructure.

Priority population – low income private tenants.

Goal: To reduce exposure to health risks associated with poor living conditions.

Intermediate indicator – to reduce the proportion of low income tenants living in substandard accommodation.

Baseline – to be derived from ABS housing survey in 1994.

stimulate inter-ministerial cooperation, regional and local public health initiatives to improve health-related living circumstances in deprived areas, and experimental interventions in deprived areas related to a range of factors such as safety from violence and urban renewal. A further five-year research programme has been agreed to develop and evaluate community interventions to reduce health problems in lower SES groups.

The National Women, Infants and Children (WIC) food supplementation programme initiated in the USA in 1973 (*see* also Chapter 10, p. 291), which combines nutritional education with a range of food supplements and healthcare access, has been shown to lengthen gestation, increase mean birth weight and reduce late fetal death.[27] The children most likely to benefit from the programme were those who were small in stature, poor, black and living in lone-parent families.

National initiatives, such as those described, are most likely to succeed in the presence of the political will and drive to tackle the problem. Where health inequalities are recognised and acknowledged, positive steps to reduce them, using intersectoral working as illustrated above, can be taken.

Local interventions

Internationally and nationally initiated projects clearly require local level intervention. The local interventions described in this section are distinguished by the fact that they are not government initiated or supported and are based on local enthusiasm and commitment to tackling health inequalities.

Accidents are one of the most important causes of injury and death in childhood and show a marked social gradient (*see* Chapter 6). Waterston describes a local initiative as part of the Healthy Cities project in Newcastle, England.[2] The model used is intersectoral, with participation of disadvantaged communities in mapping accident dangers. Parents undertook surveys to identify the absence of safe crossing points on routes to school as well as details of main roads which children needed to cross to get to school. The parents in one locality formed a 'safety-setters' injury prevention group which, among other things, raised money for home safety equipment to start a safety equipment loan scheme. The intersectoral committee is able to test out ideas with the community groups and the groups feed back information which informs the overall policy.

In the same city, an inner-city housing estate is badly served for primary healthcare services and access is a major problem.[2] An intersectoral group, including Save the Children, the local family health services authority, the social services department and the health authority, established the Family Health and Community Project. Community participation was encouraged and the views of residents sought on the main threats to health. Crime, housing and health service accessibility were identified as major problems: work was directed at upgrading houses and the local environment. There are plans to site a primary health-care facility on the estate.

A project in a poor suburb of the Belgian city of Ghent illustrates some of the difficulties of community participation.[28] Since 1981, the local medical practice had transformed itself into a multidisciplinary community health centre with participation of the local community. Community participation took the form of participation as consumers, participation in activities such as redecoration of the centre and production of the centre newsletter, and participation in policy-making, including an executive committee for the centre consisting of six patients and two health workers. However, when, in 1985, a questionnaire survey was undertaken to ascertain the level of community participation, only 13.5% said that they took part in the centre activities. These tended to be the better educated and the frequent centre users (i.e. the chronic sick). A participation model based around a health service facility which is perceived as treating the sick is likely to experience difficulties because it will be seen as relevant mainly by those who are chronically unwell and regular users rather than by those who do not regard themselves as sick.

A health authority project in the West Midlands area of England represents an interesting response to post-industrial decline in an area of traditional heavy industry. Sandwell covers a number of towns and villages in the so-called 'Black Country', west of Birmingham, which were largely dependent on the foundry industry, now in decline. Sandwell Public Health

Department set up a series of health promotion working parties, one of which – the Sandwell Economic Strategies for Health Group – addresses specifically the links between health and economic activity locally.[29] The group is charged with producing strategies related to a range of economic issues: studies of pro- and anti-health vested interests in the local economy; an unemployment strategy; an anti-poverty strategy; city planning and housing strategies; a strategy for healthy work practices, particularly in the health service itself which is a major employer. The terms of reference of the Economic Strategies for Health Group make interesting reading (Box 11.1).

The breadth of the terms of reference show an unusual commitment to a strategy for health driven by economic and social rather than medical imperatives. The elements of the anti-poverty strategy shown in Box 11.2 further illustrate this commitment.

The locally organised interventions considered above have not been vigorously evaluated. Evidence for interventions designed to reduce health inequalities is generally weak (*see* below).[30] A number of local interventions designed to reduce child health inequalities, however, have been more robustly

---

Box 11.1   Terms of reference of the Sandwell Economic Strategies for Health Study Group. (Source [29] p. 9)

1   To undertake local research on effects of work on health.
2   To undertake local research on effects of unemployment on health.
3   To advise the Health Authority on action needed in relation to unemployment and employment.
4   To advise the Health Authority on action it can take to promote healthy employment opportunities in Sandwell.
5   To advise the Health Authority on the effects of local economic strategies on health, e.g. an anti-poverty strategy.
6   To advise the Health Authority on the effects of its policies on the local economy, e.g. tobacco; food policies.
7   To advise the Health Authority on the effects of national and European policy, e.g. 1992.

Box 11.2   Some elements of an anti-poverty strategy
formulated by the Sandwell Economic Strategies for Health
Group. (Source [29] p. 9)

- Maintaining council house rents at a stable level.
- Running welfare benefits take-up campaigns.
- Funding and running: advice centres, peoples centres, family resource centre, housing project offices.
- Providing cash and help through: housing benefit, school clothing grants, education maintenance allowances, social services payments.
- Housing homeless people and providing special services for the single homeless, especially those in the 16–25 age range.
- Providing free and cheap access to leisure facilities through a 'leisure card'.
- Positively concentrating services in areas of deprivation.
- Developing 'credit unions'.
- Developing 'tenants groups'.
- Developing child care provision to enable parents to undertake further education/training and facilities for working parents.
- Setting up social services and housing 'patch' offices.
- Using statutory powers to control homes in multiple occupation.
- Providing information on loan sharks and high pressure salespeople and using statutory powers to control them.
- Food cooperatives for unemployed/low-paid workers.
- Health/social loan schemes for home and road safety equipment.

---

evaluated. An accident reduction programme in Central Harlem, based on a multi-agency Healthy Neighborhoods coalition,[31] using a 'before–after' evaluation with historical and non-randomised concurrent controls, showed a statistically significant reduction in relative risk for all target injuries and for assault. A randomised control trial of a community mothers' programme in Dublin, designed to provide home visiting by trained volunteers from the community under study,[32] showed a significant increase in uptake of immunisations in the intervention group, and mothers in this group were better on measures of tiredness and feeling miserable. In addition, both mothers and children in the intervention group had better diets.

Individual health worker interventions

Health workers may feel isolated and impotent in the face of the overwhelming odds of socio-economic influences on health. Apart from the solution of working in groups and attempting the kind of initiatives considered above, there are individual approaches which are able to alleviate and modify the effects of poverty. Addressing health visitors specifically, Blackburn makes the following assertion:

> *While health visitors cannot eradicate poverty, they can help families to avoid, mitigate and cope with the material and health effects and stresses of breadline living. It is easy to dismiss ameliorative responses as trivial, as failure to tackle the root causes of poverty. But ameliorative and preventive responses are import-ant to families. It is essential to remember that em-powering, sensitive responses at a time of continuing economic recession are better than ones that blame the victim and they can be combined with, or form part of, a strategy concerned with social change.* ([33] p. 369)

There seem to be some key elements to individual practice aimed at ameliorating the worst effects of poverty on health: sensitivity to and understanding of the structural roots of poverty – if a health worker thinks that the poor are poor because of idleness or lack of thrift then they are unlikely to be sympathetic to the problems of coping in poverty; awareness of the limitations of low income when giving advice – Blackburn states that all advice has financial and emotional costs, and advice such as 'give them fresh vegetables', 'buy a stair gate', 'take them to play group' all have costs attached to them; aware-ness of and advocacy in welfare rights are important in helping families maximise their income levels; advocacy for individual families and groups of families related to health service access and housing provision; the ability to be flexible in service delivery and to make your element of the service accessible. A further essential is a determination to break down lay–professional barriers which can get in the way of good communication and a genuine commitment to partnership with parents in the healthcare of their children.[2,15]

Paediatricians and other specialists, who in some countries traditionally practise in hospitals or privately in privileged communities, need to consider where they offer their clinical expertise and where it is likely to be most effective. Community-based consultant clinics in areas of deprivation may enable families to access specialist advice without the costs of transport and time incurred in a visit to hospital.[34]

Effectiveness of interventions

Interventions to reduce health inequalities have not been evaluated as thoroughly as many biomedical interventions. There have been two reviews of interventions designed to reduce health inequalities. Using a systematic review methodology, the NHS Centre for Reviews and Dissemination reviewed 94 studies and concluded that, despite the weakness of some of the evidence, there are interventions which the NHS can use to reduce variations in health.[30] Using a less rigorous methodology, Gepkens and Gunning-Schepers reviewed 98 evaluated studies of interventions designed to reduce health inequalities.[35] Most of these are local and many are based on traditional health-care delivery and health education. Table 11.2 summarises the effectiveness of these interventions.

Many of the health education studies claimed to have increased knowledge and to have achieved attitudinal and behavioural change, but few were shown to directly improve health outcomes in poor social and economic groups.

The projects and initiatives considered above reflect some of the principles essential to tackling health inequalities successfully. Many are not specifically health service interventions but they all include health as an important sector. Application of the principles outlined above cannot be expected to produce

Table 11.2   Tackling inequalities in health: type and effectiveness of evaluated interventions reported in the health literature. (Source [1] p. 27)

Type of intervention	Effective	Inconclusive	Ineffective	Total
Structural measures (mainly healthcare finance)	11	4	1	16
Traditional healthcare (preventive and screening services)	5	3	3	11
Health education:				
• providing information	6	6	4	16
• providing information and personal support	32	12	5	49
• health promotion and structural measures	2	1	–	3
Remainder	2	1	–	3
Total	58	27	13	98

instant results. They are most likely to succeed in a positive political climate. Those not working in such a climate should not despair: many of the examples given above show how the principles can be applied in everyday work and in new initiatives, even when working 'against the political tide'. Evaluation of projects to tackle health inequalities is difficult and remains weak.[25,30] A research agenda and commitment are needed to construct a firm scientific foundation to this work. Research directions are considered next.

Future research directions

There is a widespread feeling that knowledge of the health effects of poverty and low SES is already extensive and the focus should now be on evaluating interventions to reduce inequalities. In my view there remain a number of strong arguments for continuing to study the relationship between poverty and child health: first, socio-economic influences on health are among the most important health determinants and, compared with studies of behavioural factors such as smoking, are a neglected aspect of health research; second, current knowledge of trends in health inequalities is limited and needs to be strengthened; third, traditional measures of SES such as social or occupational class now inadequately reflect social differences in health outcomes and new measures need to be refined and tested; fourth, our knowledge of the mechanisms by which poverty and low SES influence health is poor – further work in this area is essential if we are to understand how to intervene most effectively to reduce health inequalities; fifth, the causal debate does not stand still – my account of the historical background to this debate shows that it cannot be neglected and, even when apparently won, political and economic change can rapidly undermine an apparent consensus.[13]

Studying the relationship of poverty to child health

The following areas need further study:

- child health differentials in mortality using different SES measures
- poverty and child morbidity using marker conditions
- poverty and self-reported/parent-reported illness experience in children
- poverty and self-reported health and measures of life quality
- international comparisons of health differentials and trends using common SES and health outcome measures
- equity and inequity in child health service delivery.

Mediators between poverty and health

The following areas need further study:

- models and causal pathways between poverty and child health

- specific mechanisms by which poverty influences child health

- specific mechanisms by which wealth protects against adverse health outcomes

- the role of psychosocial factors and low self-esteem in mediating the relationship between relative poverty and health in developed countries

- international comparisons of the influence of income distribution within countries on specific child health outcomes.

Evaluating interventions

The following questions need further research:

- Which interventions are effective?

- How is effectiveness to be measured?

- What are the principles and main determinants of effective interventions?

Poverty, absolute and relative, is the main determinant of child health in developing and developed countries and yet it receives relatively little medical research attention. The main focus of work on health inequalities remains health-related behaviours. It has been somewhat cynically, but truthfully, observed that poverty causes health problems of epidemic proportions and, if it were an infection that affected the rich as well as the poor, it would have been the focus of a massive research initiative to find a cure or at least a vaccine. Research programmes with their focus on health inequalities and socio-economic factors in disease causation are essential. Secondary analysis of existing longitudinal study data sets (for example the UK National Cohort Studies) using SES measures other than the Registrar General's Social Class are a potentially fruitful source of data for constructing models and causal pathways. New longitudinal studies asking new questions (for example, focusing on the role of stress and psychosocial factors in mediating between poverty and poor health outcomes) will also be needed to supplement the existing data. Health practitioners and academics need to give this area greater priority and press for increased allocation of research funding to inequalities research.

Summary

1   Health service interventions can contribute to reduction of health inequalities.

2   Principles including intersectoral work, participation and empowerment, accessibility, flexibility and advocacy seem to be important to successful interventions.

3   There are numerous examples of interventions to reduce health inequalities but a paucity of clear evidence of effectiveness.

4   Successful interventions can be carried out at international, national, local and individual practitioner level.

5   Research in the area of socio-economic influences on health has been neglected.

6   Relative to the importance of poverty and low SES as health determinants, this neglect is indefensible.

7   There is a continuing need to study the links between poverty and health, particularly the mediators through which poverty exerts its influence on health.

8   A research priority is the effectiveness of interventions.

9   A centrally funded research programme similar to that developed in the Netherlands is necessary to address all aspects of health inequalities.

References

1   Benzeval M, Judge K and Whitehead M (eds) (1995) *Tackling Inequalities in Health: an Agenda for Action*. King's Fund, London.

2   Waterston A (1995) How can child health services con-
tribute to a reduction in health inequalities in childhood? In
Progress in Community Child Health, Vol. 1 (ed. NJ Spencer).
Churchill Livingstone, London.

3   British Medical Association (1995) *Inequalities in Health*.
BMA Scientific Affairs Department, London.

4   Mackenbach JP (1995) Tackling inequalities in health. *BMJ*.
310:1152–3.

5   McIntyre L, Travers K and Dayle JB (1999) Children's feeding programs in Atlantic Canada: reducing or reproducing
inequities? *Can. J. Public Health*. 90:196–200.

6   Stagner MW and Duran MA (1997) Comprehensive community initiatives: principles, practice and lessons learned.
The Future of Children. 7:132–40.

7   Pell JP, Pell ACH, Norrie J *et al.* (2000) Effect of socio-
economic deprivation on waiting time for cardiac surgery:
retrospective cohort study. *BMJ*. 320:15–19.

8   Tsouros AD and Farrington JL (1999) Epilogue. In *Social
Determinants of Health* (eds M Marmot and RG Wilkinson).
Oxford University Press, Oxford.

9   Power C (1994) Health and social inequality in Europe.
BMJ. 308:1153–6.

10   Jolly DL (1990) *The Impact of Adversity on Child Health –
Poverty and Disadvantage*. Australian College of Paediatrics,
Parkville, Victoria.

11   Anonymous (1986) Lies, damned lies and suppressed
statistics. *BMJ*. 293:349–50.

12   Townsend P and Davidson N (1982) *Inequalities in Health:
The Black Report*. Penguin, Harmondsworth.

13   Smith GD, Blane D and Bartley M (1994) Explanations
of socio-economic differences in mortality: evidence from
Britain and elsewhere. *Eur. J. Public Health*. 4:131–44.

14 Oakley A, Rigby AS and Hickey D (1993) Women and children last? Class, health and the role of maternal and child health services. *Eur. J. Public Health.* 3:220–6.

15 Spencer NJ (1995) Partnership with parents. In *Social Paediatrics* (eds B Lindstrom and NJ Spencer). Oxford University Press, Oxford.

16 Grant J (1994) *The State of the World's Children.* Oxford University Press, New York.

17 Save the Children Fund (1995) *Towards a Children's Agenda: New Challenges for Social Development.* Save the Children, London.

18 Department of Health (1992) *The Health of the Nation: A Strategy for Health in England.* HMSO, London.

19 Department of Health (1996) *Variations in Health: What Can the Department of Health and the NHS Do?* Department of Health, London.

20 Department of Health (1998) *Our Healthier Nation: A New Contract for Health.* The Stationery Office, London.

21 Department of Health (1999) *Saving Lives: Our Healthier Nation.* The Stationery Office, London.

22 Department of Health (1999) *Reducing Health Inequalities: An Action Report.* Department of Health, London.

23 Shaw M, Dorling D, Gordon D *et al.* (1999) *The Widening Gap.* The Policy Press, University of Bristol, Bristol.

24 Whitehead M, Judge K, Hunter DJ *et al.* (1993) Tackling inequalities in health: the Australian experience. *BMJ.* 306: 783–7.

25 Mackenbach JP (1994) Socioeconomic inequalities in health in the Netherlands: impact of a five-year research programme. *BMJ.* 309:1487–91.

26   World Health Organization (1985) *Targets for Health for All*. WHO, Copenhagen.

27   Rush D, Alvir J, Johnson KS *et al.* (1988) The National WIC Evaluation: evaluation of the special supplemental food program for women, infants and children. *Am. J. Clin. Nutr.* **48**:412–28.

28   Cook J, Pechevis M and Waterston A (1995) Community diagnosis and participation. In *Social Paediatrics* (eds B Lindstrom and NJ Spencer). Oxford University Press, Oxford.

29   Middleton J (1990) Life and death in Sandwell: where public health and economic health meet. *Local Government Policy Making.* **16**:3–9.

30   NHS Centre for Reviews and Dissemination (1995) *Review of research on the effectiveness of Health Service interventions to reduce variations in health*. CRD Report 3, NHS CRD, University of York, York.

31   Davidson LL, Durkin MS, Kuhn L *et al.* (1994) The impact of the Safe Kids/Healthy Neighborhoods Injury Prevention Program in Harlem, 1988 through 1991. *Am. J. Public Health.* **84**:580–6.

32   Johnson Z, Howell F and Molloy B (1993) Community mothers' programme: randomised controlled trial of non-professional intervention in parenting. *BMJ.* **306**:1449–52.

33   Blackburn C (1991) Family poverty: what can health visitors do? *Health Visitor.* **64**:368–70.

34   Spencer NJ (1993) Consultant paediatric outreach clinics: a practical step in integration. *Arch. Dis. Child.* **68**:496–8.

35   Gepkens AR and Gunning-Schepers L (1993) *Interventions for Addressing Socioeconomic Inequalities in Health*. Institute of Social Medicine, University of Amsterdam.

12

Conclusions

In this book I have brought together evidence for the relationship between poverty and child health from a range of sources, national, international and historical. The evidence confirms that poverty and low socio-economic status have been linked with child health in all settings and all historical periods. This continuity in itself suggests a strong causal link and confirms the place of poverty as a major determinant of child health outcomes.

The book has summarised evidence for the role of social change and improvements in living standards in the dramatic improvements in health in the developed countries since the beginning of the 20th century. This is further confirmation of the causal link between poverty and low living standards and health. Equally, it illustrates the limited role played by medical treatment and medical advances in these health gains. The continued existence of diseases among children in less developed countries, for which preventive measures are fully understood and effective, is further evidence that social and environmental circumstances powerfully influence health and determine access to medical treatment and prevention. The ability of some less developed countries to eradicate these diseases by determined social and health policies and, in the process, to reduce health inequalities adds further weight to the conclusion that future improvements in health in all countries depend more on social and economic policies than medical interventions, although these can be highly effective if introduced as part of overall social and economic policies which favour the poor.

Ever since the links between poverty and health were first noted in the early part of the 19th century, there has been a fierce political debate centred on explanations for this association. Although the details of the debate have varied, and still vary according to setting, the main explanations have remained remarkably consistent across time and place. The detrimental health effects of living in poverty have been attributed, on the one hand, to the ignorance and behaviour of the poor and, on the other, to the structures of poverty and its associated disadvantages and deprivations. It is remarkable that the same debate now raging in the UK and the USA is reflected faithfully in the less developed countries, where those in poverty are castigated for their ignorance and lack of hygiene, and in the past, in today's developed countries, where the poor were held responsible through ignorance and 'fecklessness' for their health deficits.

The focus on behaviours, such as gin drinking, which was blamed for the plight of the poor in Victorian Britain, and smoking, which is currently blamed for illness among the poor, substitutes for focus on the structural elements of poverty and serves to divert attention from income disparities and the vast gulf in consumption and choice between the rich and the poor. This focus allows the blame for health inequalities to be shifted from the rich and powerful to the poor themselves. The rich are then able to continue to enjoy their advantages unencumbered by the need to address the plight of those less fortunate. With some notable exceptions, medical research has contributed to this process by its focus on disease in the individual according to the medical model and the focus on behavioural causes of adverse health outcomes. The search for a single causal factor in health outcomes has helped to distort our understanding of the complexity of the relation between health and social circumstances; there is a need to shift the research focus to exploring causal pathways which incorporate and take into account the social context of behaviour and the intimate links which tie behaviour to social and environmental circumstances.

As indicated above, the evidence I have brought together in this book has profound implications for social, economic and health policy at an international and national level as well as important implications and lessons for local and individual child health workers. There is clear evidence to link social and economic policies which increase poverty and push more people into economic vulnerability and penury, with increasing health inequalities. The converse is also true; policies which set out to reduce poverty and improve the access of the poor to health and other services are associated in less developed and developed countries with reductions in health inequalities and improvements in health outcomes for the poor.

The main conclusions of the book can be summarised as follows:

- There is a global and historical continuity linking poverty and child health.

- Poverty and child health in less developed and developed countries are causally linked.

- Relative and absolute poverty are useful concepts and both are linked with adverse child health outcomes.

- Structural explanations of child health inequalities in developed and less developed countries are more able to account for the available evidence.

- Genetic differences related to ethnic origin influence child health, but socio-economic and environmental factors are the main determinants of health differences between and within ethnic groups.

- Child health inequalities can be tackled by social, economic and health policies which are aimed at reducing income disparities and improving the access of the poor to essential services, including primary healthcare, food, water and education.

- Health services alone cannot address the health problems caused by poverty but, working imaginatively with other agencies, they can reduce health inequalities and promote equity in health.

- Child health workers who are committed to improving the health of all children can play an important role by supporting poor families and their children and working in areas where their individual contribution directly alleviates the health consequences of poverty.

- Research into the relationship between poverty and health should be strengthened with financial resources allocated specifically to a comprehensive programme exploring the mechanisms by which poverty influences health, health inequality trends and interventions, and policies which reduce health inequalities and ameliorate the adverse health effects of poverty.

Appendix: Child poverty in rich nations

This short appendix has been added to incorporate material from the UNICEF publication *A League Table of Child Poverty in Rich Nations*,[1] published in June 2000 as the second edition of this book was going to press. It provides data of particular relevance to the reasons for different levels of child poverty in rich nations and should be read as a supplement to the section *Factors underlying child poverty trends in developed countries* (Chapter 2, pp. 40–5).

Child poverty data from 23 OECD countries are examined and the key findings are summarised below:

- child poverty rates in the world's wealthiest nations vary from less than 3% to over 25%

- the UK, Italy, USA and Mexico have the highest rates of children in relative poverty (less than half the national median income)

- differences in the proportion of children living in lone-parent families have relatively little influence on the differences in child poverty rates between countries but, within each country, a child's chances of living in poverty average about four times higher in lone-parent families

- there is a close relationship between child poverty rates and the percentage of households with children in which there is no adult in work, and the percentage of full-time workers earning less than two-thirds of the national median wage

- countries with the lowest child poverty rates allocate the highest proportions of GNP to social expenditure, and differences in tax and social expenditure mean that some countries reduce child poverty by as much as 20% and others by as little as 5%

- the investment required to eliminate child poverty is relatively small amounting to 0.48% of GNP in the UK and 0.66% in the USA.

[1] UNICEF (2000) *A League Table of Child Poverty in Rich Nations*. Innocenti Report Card No.1. UNICEF, Innocenti Research Centre, Florence, Italy.

Index